# IN VIVO

T0256084

*THE CULTURAL MEDIATIONS OF BIOMEDICAL SCIENCE*

Phillip Thurtle and Robert Mitchell, Series Editors

# IN VIVO

*THE CULTURAL MEDIATIONS OF BIOMEDICAL SCIENCE*
is dedicated to the interdisciplinary study of the medical and life sciences,
with a focus on the scientific and cultural practices used to process data,
model knowledge, and communicate about biomedical science. Through
historical, artistic, media, social, and literary analysis, books in the series
seek to understand and explain the key conceptual issues that animate
and inform biomedical developments.

*THE TRANSPARENT BODY*

A Cultural Analysis of Medical Imaging

BY JOSÉ VAN DIJCK

*GENERATING BODIES AND GENDERED SELVES*

The Rhetoric of Reproduction in Early Modern England

BY EVE KELLER

# GENERATING BODIES AND GENDERED SELVES

*The Rhetoric of Reproduction in Early Modern England*

## EVE KELLER

A SAMUEL AND ALTHEA STROUM BOOK

UNIVERSITY OF WASHINGTON PRESS  SEATTLE / LONDON

This book is published with the assistance
of a grant from the Stroum Book Fund,
established through the generosity of
Samuel and Althea Stroum.

University of Washington Press
P.O. Box 50096, Seattle, WA 98145 U.S.A
www.washington.edu/uwpress

The paper used in this publication is
acid-free and 90 percent recycled from
at least 50 percent post-consumer waste.
It meets the minimum requirements of
American National Standard for Information
Sciences—Permanence of Paper for Printed
Library Materials, ANSI z39.48-1984.

Library of Congress
Cataloging-in-Publication Data

Keller, Eve, 1960–
Generating bodies and gendered selves :
the rhetoric of reproduction in early
modern England / Eve Keller.
p. ; cm. — (In vivo)
"A Samuel and Althea Stroum Book."
Includes bibliographical references and
index.
ISBN 0-295-98641-7 (pbk. : alk. paper)
1. Gynecology—England—History.
2. Human reproduction—England—
History. 3. Obstetrics—England—History
4. Gynecology—Philosophy.   I. Title.
II. Series: In vivo (Seattle, Wash.)
[DNLM: 1. Gynecology—history—
England. 2. Reproduction—England.
3. Women's Health—history—England.
WP 11 FE5 K29g 2006]
RG518.G7K45   2006
618.1′00942—dc22          2006016948

To David, Jessye, and Avir,

*whom I adore*

# CONTENTS

# MODERN MODULATIONS

# ACKNOWLEDGMENTS

I HAVE LIVED WITH THIS PROJECT FOR A LONG TIME; now that it nears completion, I am happy to acknowledge some of the debts, both personal and professional, that I have accrued along the way. Susan Greenfield has read much of the manuscript, offering insight and encouragement in equal measure; others, including Michael McVaugh, Elizabeth Harvey, Stuart Sherman, Jeffrey Masten, Catherine Weiss, and the two anonymous readers from the Press, pushed me to be both more coherent and more complete. Much of this material I have presented at various conferences of the Society for Literature, Science, and the Arts, an organization that embodies what I value most in academia: intellectual generosity, adventurous curiosity, and an abiding joy in conversation. I am grateful to all in SLSA who have helped me, especially Susan Squier and Richard Nash. SLSA also brought me to Phillip Thurtle and Robert Mitchell, editors of In Vivo, and to Jacqueline Ettinger and Dipika Nath of the University of Washington Press, all of whom warmly welcomed both me and the early modern into their vision of the series.

Three chapters in *Generating Bodies and Gendered Selves* are expanded versions of previously published essays. Chapter 4 is adapted from an essay in *Women's Studies*, pp. 131–62; © 1998, reproduced with permission of Taylor & Francis, Inc. (http://www.taylorandfrancis.com). Chapter 5 is adapted from "Embryonic Individuals: The Rhetoric of Seventeenth-Century Embryology and the Construction of Early-Modern Identity," in *Eighteenth-Century Studies*, vol. 33, no. 3, pp. 321–48; © 2000 American Society for Eighteenth-Century Studies; reprinted with permission of The Johns Hopkins University Press. Chapter 6 is adapted from "The Subject of Touch: Medical Authority in Early Modern Midwifery," originally published in *Sensible Flesh: On Touch in Early Modern Culture,* ed. Elizabeth D. Harvey (Philadelphia: University of Pennsylvania Press, 2003); reprinted by permission of the University of Pennsylvania Press.

# LIST OF ABBREVIATIONS

| | |
|---|---|
| *UP* | Galen's *On the Usefulness of the Parts of the Body* |
| *M* | Helkiah Crooke's *Microcosmographia: A Description of the Body of Man* |
| *NF* | Galen's *On the Natural Faculties* |
| *HM* | John Banister's *The Historie of Man* |
| *MA* | Nicholas Sudell's *Mulierum Amicus; or, the Woman's Friend* |
| *J.BM* | Richard Jonas's edition of *The Byrth of Mankynde* |
| *R.BM* | Thomas Raynalde's edition of *The Byrth of Mankynde* |
| *DM* | Nicholas Culpeper's *A Directory for Midwives, or A Guide for Women* |
| *PP* | Lazarus Riverius's *The Practice of Physicke* |
| *BD* | Edward Jorden's *A Briefe Discourse of a Disease Called the Suffocation of the Womb* |
| *DG* | William Harvey's *Anatomical Exercises on the Generation of Animals* |
| *PT* | *Philosophical Transactions of the Royal Society* |
| *TT* | Kenelm Digby's *Two Treatises* |
| *HG* | Nathaniel Highmore's *The History of Generation* |
| *OG* | F. J. Cole's "Dr. William Croone On Generation" |
| *IM* | Edmund Chapman's *Essay on the Improvement of Midwifery* |
| *CPM* | Sarah Stone's *A Complete Practice of Midwifery* |
| *OM* | Percival Willughby's *Observations in Midwifery* |
| *JS* | John Symcotts's *A Seventeenth-Century Doctor and His Patients* |
| *AMI* | Henry van Deventer's *The Art of Midwifery Improv'd* |
| *CM* | William Giffard's *Cases in Midwifery* |

# GENERATING BODIES AND GENDERED SELVES

# INTRODUCTION

I N THE LATE SEVENTEENTH CENTURY, THE JOURNAL
*Philosophical Transactions of the Royal Society* reported on the latest work of a
researcher in fetal osteology: having removed from a dead woman's uterus
a blood clot the size of a cherry, the gentleman was startled to discover within
the clot what he called the "first lineaments of a child." What assumptions about
the self make it possible to describe as a *child* what one sees in a mass of blood
no bigger than a cherry? Some decades earlier, William Harvey, performing empirical research on the generation of animals, had "discovered" that male semen
has no physical contact with the "egg" at conception. What concerns about the
rights of paternity might then be implied in his description of the resulting conception as "freeborn," an entity "independent" of the mother? When a physician describes the anatomy of the human womb as both "bridled" and "free,"
what understandings of woman might render reasonable so apparent a paradox? What kind of psychosomatics must govern a therapeutic regimen in which
the recommended treatment for a "misplaced" womb is to tie down not the
womb, but the woman, "so as to cause pain"?

*Generating Bodies and Gendered Selves* explores questions such as these, seeking in the rhetoric of bio-medical writing about reproduction the ideas about
selfhood that come to animate the modern period. If early modern England saw
the emergence of the modern, liberal self, it fostered equally the inception of
what became modern biological research and medical practice. The seventeenth
century in particular was also a time when English-language book publishing
began to flourish, when heavy and heady tomes of philosophical biology along
with cheap and popular books of practical physic first became widely available

3

to an unlatined audience. These diverse topics—the emergence of modern self-hood, the beginnings of modern bio-medicine, the proliferation of vernacular book publishing—have all been treated independently in the critical literature of their respective fields; it is my contention that they have much to tell us about early modern England, and about our own era as well, if considered in concert.[1]

Forging, therefore, a critical nexus among medical history, cultural studies, and literary analysis, I perform close readings of vernacular medical texts in a variety of genres—learned anatomies, commercial books of physic, midwifery manuals, collections of case histories, and published reports of medical research—in order to demonstrate the textured interrelations between discursive formulations of the body, particularly the generative body, and emerging understandings of the self in early modern England. In an age marked by social, intellectual, and political upheaval, early modern bio-medicine, I argue, inscribes in the flesh and the functioning of the bodies it produces the manifold questions about gender relations, political organization, and philosophical positioning that together give rise to the modern western liberal subject.

■ It is perhaps a sign of our desired dissociation from its legacy that we now seem able to describe so readily the network of ideas about personhood that anchors western modernity. Though variously articulated over the past 350 years, these ideas hold that personhood consists of an individuated and autonomous core self, one that is reflexively aware, self-determining, and agential. This self is furthermore imbued with a rich (if not wholly conscious) interiority that is conceived of as inhabiting or possessing a body rather than being coextensive with one. Above all, this self is understood to precede social formation and is deemed both natural and universal to human being. In their manifold forms, these ideas of human being found the legitimacy of liberal democratic freedom and rights, of contractual government and market capitalism; a version of them is elaborated in most forms of psychoanalysis; and, perhaps paradoxically, they currently animate both sides of the abortion debate, pitting a fetus's "right to life" against a woman's "right to choose." Though once premised as being constant across time and cultures, these notions of personhood are now recognized to be decidedly bounded historical constructs, finding their most specific and grounding articulation in the early modern period. One can see their varying contours in Hobbes's derivation of political right and duty from the self-interest of autonomous individuals; in Locke's argument that the continuity of persons inheres in the continuity of consciousness; and, perhaps preeminently, in the characteristics of the Cartesian cogito, the self that exists exclusively as an unextended thinking thing, different in essence from material, extended being—an idea integral to the Cartesian Enlightenment if not to Descartes himself.

In the past few decades, studies and critiques of the emergence of these notions of personhood have become prominent in explorations of the literature, politics, philosophies, and theologies of the early modern period.[2] But as much as the history of modern subjectivity has been of critical concern across numerous disciplines, the participation of bio-medical literature in the generation and proliferation of these ideas has been rather less examined. This relative neglect is currently being corrected; in the past, however, it resulted less from a reasoned assessment of the importance of bio-medical literature to the emergence of modern selfhood than from a tradition of historical scholarship that tended to pursue different kinds of questions.

A hundred years ago, the prevailing evolutionary model of history in science and medicine deemed a *true* history to consist of the description and analysis of only those specific discoveries that could be said to lead progressively to the current state of the field; the cultural conditions of *making* those discoveries were discounted as inessential additions to, or presuppositions of, the discoveries themselves. This style of doing history has been considered methodologically suspect since at least the 1930s and the emphasis has since shifted from the mapping of *progress* to more expansive explorations of the making of medical knowledge and the social history of medicine. These concerns have generated studies that, instead of focusing on the great figures and important discoveries of medicine, turn their attention to "history from below," analyzing, for example, the medical marketplace, the varied cultures of medical practice, and the textured experience of the patient.[3]

In the social history of medicine, two recently published works by early modern historians suggest the interpretive possibilities of broad cultural analyses of the reproductive body. The first, Mary Fissell's *Vernacular Bodies*, explores "ordinary people's" ideas about the body by examining all manner of "cheap print"—that is, the small books, broadsides, and pamphlets that were available to practically anyone who could read.[4] Concerned chiefly with what these cheap print texts say about reproduction and the reproductive body in the context of the Protestant Reformation and the English civil wars, Fissell argues that people's ideas about reproduction modeled larger questions of gender relations and politics that were keenly at issue at the time. Lisa Cody's *Birthing the Nation* treats a later period, focusing on how the gradual emergence of male authority over sex and birth during the long eighteenth century was intricately bound up with the formation of national, religious, and gendered identities.[5] Both these studies are interdisciplinary in scope, charting their investigations of the body's many meanings through texts and events—such as popular ballads and bawdy jokes or more sober legislation about out-of-wedlock motherhood—that have generally not been included in traditional medical or intellectual histories of their periods. Though neither focuses exclusively on bio-medical literature, nor specifically treats the engagement of bio-medicine in the formation of models of gendered subjectivity, these works together suggest a growing awareness of and interest in the ways in which biology and medical practice in the early modern period both incorporate and enable larger cultural concerns about gender.[6]

Some early modern literary scholars, too, have explored the bio-medical literature of the period, prompted in large part by Thomas Laqueur's influential study of the "making" of sex "from the Greeks to Freud."[7] Generally, though, literary scholars have mined this material as a means of elucidating cultural norms or as an aid in illuminating more traditionally literary texts rather than as primary texts in their own right.[8] In a recent and impressive collection of essays called *Reading the Early Modern Passions*, for example, a number of prominent literary scholars turn to a particular sourcebook of Renaissance psychology, Thomas Wright's 1604 medical handbook *The Passions of the Mind in General*, to explain and exemplify early modern understandings of material psychology.[9] As one of the authors puts it, Wright's handbook offers "puzzled modern readers some help" in understanding how thoroughly embodied the early modern psyche was.[10] Wright's handbook serves as a means of explanation and elucidation but not as a text *itself* to be explained and elucidated. There are, of course, exceptions to this pattern—in some of Elizabeth Harvey's work, for example[11]—but it remains the general tendency among literary historians to incorporate medical texts into their efforts as aids to study rather than as objects of study in themselves.

What I propose in *Generating Bodies and Gendered Selves* is to combine and adapt aspects of the different approaches taken by medical and social historians on the one hand and literary scholars and critics on the other. Specifically, I engage the biological and medical texts of the period as my primary objects of study, but I read the prose patterns of those texts as rhetorical constructs. I subject the language of English bio-medicine to the kinds of close reading more commonly performed on texts traditionally considered literary, thereby hoping to tease out the texts' implicit assumptions about emerging models of personhood. To read these medical texts closely is to read them symptomatically, as early modern medical men read the body itself, marking among discernable surface patterns the signs that point to the implicit workings of a system.

Methodologically, then, one of the assumptions guiding this work is that rhetorical analysis is one way to get at what Ludwik Fleck called the "thought-styles" of a community: the non-empirical, non-conscious intellectual formulations that constitute the conceptual apparatus for perceiving and articulating ideas in science and medicine. Working against the assertions of the Vienna Circle scholars that the facts of science exist independently of any cultural impingements, Fleck pointed out, decades before Thomas Kuhn and the formalized idea of the social construction of science, that natural phenomena can be identified only in the context of conceptual frameworks that make it possible to perceive them *as* phenomena. A fact can *exist as a fact* only in the context of some language used to state it, and this language, Fleck proposed, is as much a constitutive aspect of the fact as the empirical experience that prompted its discovery in the first place.[12] Fleck's notion of a thought-style is rather more restrictive than my use of it here; for Fleck, a thought-style is specifically tied to what he called a "thought-collective," an identifiable community of working scientists whose shared assumptions make possible, both methodologically and intellectually, the work they pursue and the knowledge they produce. My sense is at once broader and simpler: I intend by the term the conceptual template that makes perception possible, the mindset that contours and colors both what one perceives and how one expresses that perception.[13] At the broadest level, *Generating Bodies and Gendered Selves* proposes that newly emerging and gendered models of the self were integral to the overarching thought-style that shaped apprehensions of the early modern body.

■ It is common these days to call for attention to the body in explorations of the self, to delineate a fully corporealized subjectivity. This is perhaps a distinctly Foucauldian inheritance, since it was primarily Foucault's work that spotlighted the ways in which the body, rather than some unfettered consciousness, constituted the true site for the social production of modern subjectivity. But it is typical, too, of much work that departs from Foucault's masculinist stance, and is particularly evident in current feminist work of scholars such as Elizabeth Grosz and Elizabeth Wilson, who have grown uncomfortable with the dismissal of the biological as untheorizable and deterministic.[14] A robust reengagement of the biological body animates Grosz's call for a "corporeal feminism" that understands the body as "the very 'stuff' of subjectivity," as it does Wilson's feminist project to "rethink our reflexive critical recoil from neurological theories of the psyche."[15] It is also explicit in the underwriting claim of modern neurophilosophy (as I will explore in chapter 1) that it is now not only possible but necessary to pursue philosophical studies of consciousness and the mind—key components in western understandings of the self—by working from the wholly material basis of the brain. These efforts, both theoretical and empirical, do not mark a return to an older style of analysis that separated the facts of nature from the constructions of culture, they do not posit the biological body as outside the contested fora of political or philosophical debate; rather, they engage the biological body in its material detail as a participant in the debates themselves. Wilson, for example, studies neuroscience specifically as "an arena of politically useful perspectives for feminism."[16] Simply put, explorations of the self must take the material body into account.

But the association between the body and the self works from the other direction, too: the body, and writing about the body, always assumes, if only implicitly, some understandings of the self. Shigehisa Kuriyama has shown, elegantly and elaborately, how the systems of ancient Chinese and Greek medicine imagined human bodies, and thereby human being in the world, in startlingly different ways. Whereas the Greeks understood muscles as the conduits for voluntary action, for example, the Chinese did not even have a word to indicate what we call "muscle"; they pictured the body instead in terms of the tracts and sites of acupuncture. Ancient notions of personhood, Kuriyama contends, align with these divergent somatic visions: the Greek concern with agency and will, manifest in muscle, contrasts against the Chinese aspiration for proper flow and healthful emptiness, manifest in the subtle movement of the chi.[17]

Closer to the concerns of this study, the overlap between formulations of body and self can be seen in William Harvey's work on the circulation of the blood. Harvey's proposal that blood moves through the body in a closed circuit contravened not only Galenic anatomy but also Galenic understandings of the person. Once the blood was seen to circulate in a closed somatic system and the vital spirit, which animates the blood, was understood to be an aspect of the blood itself rather than something elaborated in the blood from respired air, the organism was newly severed from its ambient environment: the closing of the body, its self-sustaining autonomy, parallels the emerging autonomy of the liberal self.[18]

The relation between body- and self-constructs is even sometimes accessible by pressing on the shifting meanings of single words. In ancient Greek medicine, for example, the word *organon* indicated not, as *organ* does for us, simply a part that performs a function. Rather, *organon* indicated an instrument, a tool. Organs were body parts designed to carry out the acts of the soul, such as seeing or breathing; the body's organs, as the body itself, were designed to carry out the purposive actions of the soul. As Galen explained, "The usefulness of all the organs is related to the soul. For the body is the instrument of the soul, and . . . is adapted to the character and faculties of the soul."[19] Galen was ambivalent about the order of priority here, even writing a treatise to demonstrate the opposite, namely, that the soul follows or depends on the temperament of the body.[20] But the inextricability of organ and soul, soma and psyche, bespeaks a sense of self far different from an anatomy that envisions organs solely as functional parts of a body that do not work on behalf of anything else.

■  Although concerned with the medically conceived body as a whole, *Generating Bodies and Gendered Selves* focuses specifically on the generating body for both historical and conceptual reasons. In the early modern period, the bio-medicine of generation was changing in both theory and practice, really for the first time in well over a millennium. It is at this point of change that we can see the first signs of a truly modern bio-medicine. In the realm of medical theory, as chapters 4 and 5 will show, the late sixteenth and the seventeenth centuries saw the first studies in developmental embryology since Aristotle; no longer a static field of description, embryology turned to the systematic study of the course of development of an animal, charting on a daily basis the changes that transform an undifferentiated mass into a living organism.[21] In practical medicine, as chapter 6 explores, the late seventeenth and early eighteenth centuries saw both the first consistent entrance of men into the birthing room and the development of new techniques for handling births; the period thus marks the beginning of what came to be called obstetrics.

But there are conceptual reasons as well for studying ideas of personhood in relation to the generative body. The model of the human person constructed by the liberal humanist tradition is distinctly masculine, its details typically defined through its opposition to the female; yet what constitutes the female bio-medically has been a rather contested issue. From classical through medieval times, authorities debated whether *woman* was better defined specifically by the womb and its generative capacities, or more generally by her overall somatic constitution, that is, by her colder, moister temperament. But increasingly in the later Middle Ages and in the early modern period, woman grew more tightly identified with her generative function, and women's healthcare increasingly became allied with the medical concerns of childbearing.[22] As medical literature in this period worked to consolidate a notion of modern man, it did so in opposition to a notion of modern woman, and woman was defined by her generative function. Accordingly, texts engaged with questions of generation—its theory, physiology, anatomy, and the practice of what we call gynecology and obstetrics—are appropriate sites to explore questions relating to what I will claim are distinctly gendered models of personhood.

I thus rely in my analysis on what is now a critical commonplace—that the early modern self is never constructed in isolation, is never an autonomous discovery of the unencumbered intellect. Rather, it is always and inevitably deployed in relation to, really in contrast to, some posited opposition. At the simplest level, that opposition enables its definition, that is, we know something is *x* because it is opposed to *not-x*; in this case, for example, rational because opposed to irrational, or mindful because opposed to embodied. But the oppositions, which are necessary to ground the identifying characteristics of a model, are not precise, and they are never entire. For even as it seeks to define itself against an asserted opposition, the model always participates to some extent in what it endeavors to oppose. The clearest example of this paradoxical maneuver appears in the last chapter of this book, in which the heroics of modern medicine, exemplified in the rational efficiency of the male midwife, establish the supremacy of mind over matter by employing precisely what the model seeks to devalue, that is, manual—material—interventions in birth. But versions of this paradox are repeatedly evident in the works I treat. In chapter 2, I describe how the embodied psychophysiology of ancient bio-medicine is revived in the early modern period to serve as a model of masculine selfhood that actually eschews embodiment. In chapters 4 and 5, I describe how, for the first time in western history, contemporary research in embryology grants subjectivity to embryos; in doing so it promotes the idea of masculine self-determination as a given of nature, but the model emerges only as a rhetorical response to a range of perceived threats to masculine authority.

Foundational in all these incomplete efforts at opposition is the female, in her anatomy, physiology, reproductive function, and parturient experience. The idea of the early modern person in these texts is always erected in contrast to her. But even this is a fraught effort because the female itself is not a univocal category; rather, importantly, if not surprisingly, the female is an unstable, fluctuating, troubled ground, and the contours of her contradictoriness show up the problems of the masculine models themselves. For the female, in her anatomy (whether human or animal), in her generative capacity, in her position as parturient patient, is ever and again presented as not a single thing but as the meeting point of opposites, as both agential and passive, as embodied subject and as only body, as self-willing and silent. The female occupies an ambivalent space: at once a subject and subjected, characterized, for example, by a womb that is described as literally, physically "free," but then figuratively as free only to the extent that it—the womb itself—consents, freely, to its subjugation to a female's reproductive role.

I therefore think it inaccurate to suggest that the ideology of gender animating early modern bio-medicine is built on exact, hierarchical binaries. Though easy oppositions do, at times, emerge (as, for example in popular renderings of an enlivened male fetus posturing within a clearly inert and dislocated womb), the dichotomies in general are not nearly so neat[23] (see plate 4, page 77). In a variety of ways, bio-medicine did align the female with characteristics of universal Man. Birth was frequently assumed to result from the joint efforts of the female and the fetus, for example, so that a childbearing woman was considered to be fully a participant in the process of labor and delivery.[24] In one important embryological text of the period, the female is even considered "the stronger party in generation."[25] The point, however, is that the portrait is not consistent: the female is a participatory, possessive, agential subject, but *not always*, and never completely. The rhetoric always undermines the coherence of the construct.

This ambivalence points to the tensions in the model of male personhood that these texts promote; it claims to be universal but is not; it seems to be achieved by empirical research and reasoned analysis but is more deeply designed by rhetorical tropes. The story I tell is, therefore, not one of the gradual emergence and subsequent demise of a singular notion of the self; it is not a story that progresses from stability to crisis, from modern discovery to postmodern deconstruction. Rather, it is a story of emergence uneasily dependent upon and not completely sustained by the contradictoriness of what it endeavors to define itself against, namely, the generative body of the female.

■ It is important to understand that in tracing the connections between early modern bio-medical literature and the generation of gendered subjectivity I am not proposing a single, unitary model, either of the body or of the self. That concepts of the body and the self are historically and culturally specific is perhaps the primary animating insight of current critiques of the liberal humanist tradition. The idea that the modern subject is not the simple discovery of progressively rational humankind but is erected in the service of very specific cultural practices—market capitalism, for example, or domestic patriarchy—binds the model of modern man to particular times and places. Thirty years ago, Clifford Geertz encouraged a cross-cultural anthropology to demonstrate precisely this lesson: the "western conception of the person," he wrote, "as a bounded, unique, more or less integrated motivational and cognitive universe, a dynamic center of awareness, emotion, judgement and action, organized into a distinctive whole and set contrastively against other such wholes and against a social and natural background is, however incorrigible it may seem to us, a rather peculiar idea within the context of the world's cultures."[26] More recently, Kuriyama undertook his comparative study of ancient and opposing bio-medical traditions to foster a similar realization: "comparative inquiry into the history of the body invites us, and indeed compels us, ceaselessly to reassess our own habits of perceiving and feeling, and to imagine alternative possibilities of being."[27]

The cultural-historical specificity of body- and self-constructs is evident, too, in the terms we use to point to personhood. The Greeks had no word reasonably translatable as *self*; the word *psyche*, typically translated as *soul*, bears in Greco-Roman medicine none of the specifically religious overtones that it does in a Christianized context. The very term *self* did not achieve currency in English until the mid-seventeenth century, and even then its connotations were more capacious than current ones, suggesting, typically in a religious context, a willful turning away from the divine, an illogical absorption in the particular over the universal, rather than what for us might be a more purely positive capacity for interiority or reflexive inquiry.[28] If Locke's understanding of personhood was innovative, it was also in the late seventeenth century still considered alarming because it severed the connection between personhood and the Christian cosmos, substituting for that connection an idea of the continuity of an isolated and individual consciousness over time.[29] Even the word *individual* retained in the seventeenth century some its Latinate meaning of "undivided," as Milton's Adam in *Paradise Lost* claims Eve as his "individual solace dear" and thus initiates a relationship that turns precisely on the changing meanings of that difficult word.[30]

As much as the contextual specificity of both body- and self-constructs is widely acknowledged, it is also important to recognize that these models are never monolithic, even within particular cultures and at particular times. To talk of the liberal humanist subject is to employ a generalization of convenience, one that provides a broad framework within which one may examine the historical specificities of its emergence. But it *is* a generalization, an instrument of analysis, rather than an accurate, monotonic picture of a period. The models of selfhood under discussion here were challenged even from their earliest formulations. Hume, for example, famously worried about his inability to catch a self separate from any particular act of cognition or perception; he doubted, in other words, precisely the idea of a stable, separable self inherent to man. Locke's entertaining of the possibility that God could give the power of thought to material substance initiated a host of eighteenth-century commentaries on the monistic ideal of thinking matter, thereby rejecting Cartesian dualism of substance.[31] And more generally still, the Enlightenment itself, so typically associated with the Cartesian cogito, with the supremacy of autonomous, rational Man, is also an era deeply suspicious of disembodiment, fearful of patterns that might presage a return to the frightful and superstitious zeal of the Puritans.[32]

Fleck's notion of a thought-style expresses this multiplicity well; thought-styles are tied more to the communities that engage them, that see and think with them, than they are to particular time periods. Thus we could say, for example, that in the first half of the seventeenth century three overlapping but distinct thought-styles vied for precedence in the midst of Galenism's decline—vitalism, mechanism, and mystical alchemy. In an important book on the discovery and gradual acceptance of the circulation of the blood, Thomas Fuchs has shown how Harvey's description of the discovery, which itself, as he says, "unhinged" Galenic physiology, was far from offering a new, revolutionary thought-style for understanding it. Harvey himself incorporated his discovery into a modified but still thoroughly vitalist physiology, and the first proponents of the new fact of the circulation were specifically those who could incorporate it into already developed systems, for example, Robert Fludd, who wrote about the circulation in the context of his mystical-alchemical understandings, and Descartes, who, much more influentially, adopted the circulation into his understanding of the mechanism of matter.[33]

In bio-medical literature dealing with generation, we find that texts differing in fundamental ways—in terms of subject matter, methodology, and philosophical commitment—all work in one way or another to promote some aspect of the gendered personhood I am sketching here. Thus, a learned text deeply entrenched in the ancient traditions of Galenism nonetheless manages to promote a modern notion of a masculine person *possessed* of body parts just as much as pioneering research in embryology promotes modern notions of self-determining volitional man. Within the field of embryology itself, texts committed to mutually exclusive philosophical outlooks, that is, committed either to vital-ist or mechanist modes of explanation, nonetheless conspire to create the mod-ern masculine subject in opposition to the feminine, suggesting that the need to promote certain understandings of personhood was more pressing, more fun-damental in early modern culture, than a writer's specific philosophical orien-tation or a genre's specific conventions. Learned no less than popular, original no less than derivative, English-language bio-medical texts of the early modern period deploy a rhetoric that grants modern selfhood to normative Man.

The models of gendered subjectivity I explore here were thus becoming part of a perspective that grew increasingly dominant over the course of the seven-teenth century. These models made the body intelligible to those who wrote about it, regardless of their differently developed and articulated philosophical, method-ological, or professional positions. My argument, then, is that emerging models of gendered subjectivity were important aspects of the bio-medical thought-styles of early modern England—they enabled apprehension of the body and unified the body's articulation across theoretical, professional, and generic divides.

■ One way to approach the particularity of early modern formulations of body and self is to set them in relation to our own, present-day concerns about embod-iment and personhood. At the turn of the twenty-first century, questions of cor-poreality and selfhood are explicitly addressed in numerous scientific and cultural-historical fields, though perhaps most noticeably in robotics and neu-rophilosophy. What happens to the idea of the human person when a promi-nent roboticist projects the possible downloading of human consciousness into a machine?[34] Is the resulting thing a human-machine hybrid, a cyborg? Is it *you* who gets downloaded into silicon circuitry? Are you still *you* when flesh is replaced by metal? Does personhood inhere in consciousness or, even more broadly, in *mind*? It is a centuries-old question, surely, but one given an edge by the advent of humanoid robotics.

Some contend that we have always been cyborgs in some ways, that we have always incorporated tools and technologies into our senses of our selves, and recent neurological imaging studies seem actually to bear this out, at least for certain primates. Experiments conducted on macaque monkeys have demon-strated that an animal will seamlessly incorporate the tools it uses into its men-tal representations of its body. For example, when a monkey is trained repeatedly to use a rake to pull food to itself, its mental map of its body—its body schema, its brain-made representation of its body—includes the space taken up not only by its arm but by the rake as well: the monkey's brain seems to represent the monkey's somatic self as a single amalgam of body and tool.[35] If one permits the conceptual leap to humans, is it valid then to say that, neurologically at least, *I* am constituted by my body and its routine extensions (glasses, prosthetic limbs, cars, pens)?

As many have commented, these questions matter in ways much more immediate and more politically pressing than academic philosophizing is considered to be. Within the western liberal humanist tradition, a tradition built over the last 250 years on the assumed existence of individual, autonomous persons each endowed with inalienable rights, how are we to determine the appropriate disbursement of rights? If persons are already cyborgs and if cyborgs are then persons, are they, too, individuals and autonomous? Do they too enjoy, for example, the right to life, liberty, and the pursuit of happiness?[36] And if neurology is now able to speak directly and empirically to questions more traditionally considered within the purview of philosophy, do we need to adjust our understanding of personhood to neurobiology's dictates?

*Generating Bodies and Gendered Selves* begins with a brief exploration of some of these questions as they arise in recent work in robotics and neurophilosophy, partly to instantiate the claim that questions of personhood are always enmeshed with questions of the body, even when the bodies in question are made of metal. But more importantly I begin with what has been called the posthuman in order to propose a series of similarities between it and the premodern, Galenic version of embodied selfhood.[37] These affinities matter because they characterize the precise points from which the early modern versions of body and self diverge: whereas both posthumanist theory and Galenism envision personhood as embodied, embedded in material context, and manifest in distributed somatic function, the early modern models by contrast strive to be disembodied, free of material constraint, and localized in the mind. The areas of affinity between the premodern and the posthuman, then, not only constitute a thread of continuity in western understandings of body and self, but also show that the models of selfhood implicated in early modern vernacular bio-medicine are in fact quite aberrant when considered from the wide perspective of western history.

After an introductory chapter that brackets the early modern between the Galenic and the posthuman, *Generating Bodies and Gendered Selves* pursues its topic in a variety of genres common to early modern medicine. The book is divided roughly in half, each part devoted to one touchstone text as well as to many lesser-known medical writings. The first section focuses on early modern renderings and revisions of ancient medicine, primarily of Galenism but also of the tradition that derived from Soranus, the second-century physician traditionally considered to have authored a gynecological text that formed the basis of the first dedicated gynecological treatises in England. Chapter 2 focuses on a major work of philosophical bio-medicine, Helkiah Crooke's *Microcosmographia*, the first and last great effort in English to systematize and update Galenism. I show how Crooke's rhetorical formulations, defying the logic of Galen's embodied psychophysiology, posit for the normative body a supervening, separable self that oversees all physical function. I further demonstrate that the normative body, and the model of selfhood it promotes, is exclusively male because the rhetoric Crooke employs to describe the female body subsumes any sense of a self within the willful workings of the womb. Pursuing the portrait of the specifically female, chapter 3 turns to a series of women's healthcare manuals, spanning roughly the century between 1550 and 1650, to elucidate the conflicted and anxious renderings of medical knowledge about women; from concerns about readership to recommendations for therapeutics, these books demonstrate the impossibility of "fixing" a female self, unless it is conceived as a womb.

The second section of the book turns to texts that treat original research and new methods of practice from the mid-seventeenth to the early eighteenth century; two chapters discuss embryology in particular. Chapter 4 offers a close reading of Harvey's *De generatione animalium* (published in 1651 and translated into English in 1653), examining how Harvey negotiates the challenges to the idea of paternity, and by extension, to the political legitimacy of patriarchy, presented by his erroneous embryological "discovery" that the semen has no physical contact with the "egg" at conception. Chapter 5 uses reports subsequently published in *Philosophical Transactions of the Royal Society* to explore how the increasing reliance on mechanist (over vitalist) explanations of embryogenesis gave rise to the historically unprecedented attribution of subjectivity to embryos.

The final chapter of the book studies the subject status accorded to the medical practitioners who specialized in childbirth and who are the forebears of what became known as obstetrics. Working with case histories written at a time when men first entered the field of midwifery, I demonstrate how the rhetorical deployment of the male midwife's *body* paradoxically established him as the exclusive *rational* authority in the birthing room—at once eclipsing the subjectivity of competing practitioners and reducing the parturient woman to silence. The male midwife in these texts epitomizes the model of male subjectivity whose generation this book studies: born in rhetoric from the body of the childbearing woman, he emerges as the paradigmatic Enlightenment hero, a self-directed, rationally ordered, thoroughly modern individual.

■   In tracing the relation between generating bodies and gendered selves in early modern England, this study raises questions of causal connection. What roles did bio-medical literature play, socially, culturally, conceptually, ideologically, in the generation of particular subjectivities? It is tempting, I think, but inaccurate, to argue that the bio-medical texts I explore helped to naturalize or normalize already entrenched social arrangements, as if appeals to the givenness, the objective self-evidence of the body, could legitimate the constructed arrangements of a culture. First of all, and perhaps most simply, it is questionable whether either medicine itself or any of its practitioners during the early modern period had the cultural authority to constitute a convincing appeal. Most medical practitioners were not trained at university, and, though their patients certainly accepted their remedies (with the general understanding that the more potent the remedy the better), they were not automatically assumed to have privileged access to knowledge. It was precisely to generate such a reputation that the medical case histories I explore in chapter 6 were so deftly designed. Second, and somewhat more subtly, nature itself was not, or was only just beginning to be, considered a neutral arbiter of cultural dispute. There was no sense, in the early modern period, as there was, for example, in the Victorian period, that a value-free natural order grounded the distinct social roles assigned to men and women. Bio-medical knowledge was simply not thought to be outside questions of cultural organization, whether those questions dealt with gender roles, political structures, or theological positions.[38] Bio-medical truths were richly imbued with signification and value; bio-medicine was a place where questions of identity, of selfhood, of human being, were worried and worked out, as they were equally, if variously, in drama, poetry, theology, law, and politics. To say this is not to unmask some ideology secretly at work, to declare that what passes for truth is constructed by hidden causalities or structures of power, or that the history of the body, studied from a perspective strictly internal to the history of medicine, is startlingly affected by factors external to it. It is, rather, to erase altogether the internal/external divide and the sense of linear causality that that divide assumes. It is a simple recognition of how thoroughly interwoven the body was with all aspects of creation, how inextricably it was entangled in a network of connections that encompassed equally the constituents of matter and the incarnation of the divine. The body was less a given, an object bearing the force of self-evidence, than something more nearly akin to what Bruno Latour has struggled to call not a matter of fact, but a "matter of concern," "an ingathering of meaning."[39]

Perhaps the preeminent contemporary theorist of science studies, Latour now finds himself wanting to evaluate the fruits of decades of social critique. In a recently published article, Latour says that it was a mistake to believe that the only way to critique matters of fact was by "moving *away* from them and directing one's attention *toward* the conditions that made them possible."[40] This, he recognizes in retrospect, had the unhappy effect of seeming to relativize the objects under study, making possible a host of unsavory alliances—for example, with neoconservative strategists who promote the "*lack of scientific certainty*" as a means of avoiding global warming legislation.[41] Taken aback by what has become of critique, Latour encourages a return to realism, but to a full-bodied, thick-description realism, in which what are accepted as matters of fact are seen as "only very partial . . . and very polemical, very political renderings" of a much broader, much more complex and "entangled" arena, which he calls "matters of concern." Under this heading he proposes to "reconnect scientific objects with their aura, their crown, their web of associations," to "accompany them back to their gathering," not thereby "to weaken them, but precisely to strengthen their claim to reality."[42]

Considering in 1929 what he called "the crisis of 'reality,'" Fleck asked, "Of what ought the absolute reality to be independent? If one wished it to be independent of man, one ought to consider that in this event it would also be of no use to man."[43] Seventy-five years later, Latour casts the same net in which to catch what is real, but casts it wider and farther and thereby reaches back to what was always a truth before we ever pretended to be modern: "Give me one matter of concern and I will show you the whole earth and heavens that have to be gathered to hold it firmly in place."[44]

*Generating Bodies and Gendered Selves* is an effort to show the bio-medical bodies of early modern England as just such matters of concern, permuted into prose through the inchoate, emerging thought-styles of modern and gendered subjectivity.

# 1 / On Either Side of the Early Modern:

## Posthuman and Premodern Bodies and Selves

INTEND TO DISCUSS A WIDE RANGE OF ENGLISH-language medical texts written between the mid-sixteenth and the early eighteenth centuries. By offering close readings of their rhetorical practices, I hope to elucidate some of the ways in which emerging understandings of gender-defined subjectivity are implicated in and enable discursive formulations of the body. But I want to begin by looking away from my subject in two, opposite directions, to the long before and the long after, because I think that considering the bio-medical versions of the early modern body in the diachronic perspective of the long arc of western intellectual history will help us to understand what is so peculiar about the bodies and selves that get constructed in the early modern period itself.

There are, of course, dangers in making the comparison I am about to propose; minimally I lay myself open to charges of presentism (that is, of anachronistically employing current conceptual categories to talk about premodern constructs) and, more generally, to the charge that I ignore crucial differences in order to make a claim about similarity. I would respond by saying that my intent is not to argue that the distant past is best understood in terms of present concerns and concepts or that ancient ideas fit easily and accurately into current preoccupations, but rather to suggest the existence of long-term and fairly broad-based continuities even amidst the epistemic upheavals of millennia. Differences abound, but there are points of contact, too, and I think they are worth noting, partly because they might help us think through questions about bodies and selves in our own time, but also, and more particularly for my purposes, because they might help us better understand how the versions of body and self that emerged in the early modern period differed from both what had gone before and what has followed since. I will argue that it is at just those points of difference, registered in the subtle rhetorical moves of these vernacular texts, that we can most clearly see what interested—and troubled—early modern writers about the idea of a self and how it might (or might not) be related to the material stuff of the bodies they wrote about.

My premise is twofold: first, that despite important and evident differences both in biological detail and in ideological and methodological assumption, there are remarkable (though typically unremarked) areas of overlap between some recent figurations of the so-called posthuman and the premodern human as it is modeled in some of the foundational medical writings of Galen; and second, that the early modern figurations of the human that this book will address differ from both the before and the after on precisely these points of overlap.

Because it offers an argument about similarity, this chapter proceeds somewhat schematically. I begin my case about these areas of overlap by establishing some of the essential characteristics of posthumanism. Although typical treatments of the posthuman emphasize the idea of the interfacing of flesh and wire, human and machine, I argue here that the underlying idea of posthumanism is broader than that. Specifically, by looking to some recent research in robotics and neurophilosophy, I point to three recurrent features of the posthuman self, namely, embodiment (the self is inextricable from its material substrate); embeddedness (the self is not an inviolable entity but rather a point in a network of relations); and distributed function (there is no homunculus or central control feature of human being; the self arises, rather, from the distributed functioning of semiautonomous systems).

Having established my portrait of the posthuman, I turn to survey some of Galen's essential ideas about physiology in order to show how these three features of posthumanism—embodiment, embeddedness, and distributed function—characterize the Galenic notion of personhood as well. I consider by turns Galen's theory of the elements to explicate his understanding of embeddedness, his views on the status and physiological role of the psyche to elucidate his position on embodiment, and his treatment of the four natural faculties to show how personhood is not separable from but consonant with the distributed workings of these psychophysiological functions. In concluding the chapter, I consider the importance of the comparison: the early modern models of selfhood with which this book is primarily concerned constitute the one clear break in otherwise continuous understandings of body and self between the premodern and the posthuman in western thought.

■  Arising from the challenges presented to the idea of human being by research and technological developments in artificial intelligence, bioengineering, and robotics, the posthuman refers to a loosely defined network of ideas about subjectivity and its relation to embodiment, agency, and information. Posthuman critiques typically treat the technoscientific—the cyborgian mergings and biological manipulations made possible in thought or practice by robotics, virtual reality, genetic engineering, and stem cell research. The posthuman cyborg is not only the person with the cochlear implant, the runner with the robotic prosthetic leg, but also the bioengineered skin graft, the laboratory-synthesized liver.[1] Wholly a hybrid, a merging of categories popularly held distinct, the posthuman tests the limits of *the human*, questioning its coherence as a category, its givenness in nature. The posthuman is therefore *post* not only in the sense of coming *after* the humanist vision but also in the sense of challenging its basic assumptions of the human self as natural, inviolable, autonomous.

Yet, as many have noted, posthumanism often perpetuates the very humanism it purports to supplant.[2] In many of its forms—though not in the one that will concern me here—posthumanism occludes the body as much as any dualism might; what counts in these versions is not the material substrate of mentality but the structure of the informational flow that results in cognitive capacity. The key idea in these versions is that the mind (whether human or artificial) can be profitably understood and analyzed as an information-processing system; as the neurophilosopher Patricia Churchland rather felicitously (if derisively) explains it, in this view, "the mind is analogous to software running on a computer. Like Adobe Photoshop, the cognitive program can be run on computers with very different hardware configurations. Consequently, although mind software can be run on the brain, it can also run on a device made of silicon chips or Jupiter goo."[3] Because the particular matter of which the creature is made is deemed incidental to its intelligence, some researchers who support this view speak comfortably of a *postbiological* future for human being. The roboticist Hans Moravec, perhaps the most notable proponent of this position, forecasts a time when it will be possible to "download" an individual's consciousness into a machine, thereby perpetuating "life"—and the individual herself—in a silicon-based, rather than a carbon-based, entity.[4] As the cultural and literary critic Katherine Hayles has pointed out, these versions of the posthuman, though radical in their belief in the possibility of a seamless interface between human being and intelligent machine, actually perpetuate one of the central features of liberal humanist subjectivity, namely, the privileging of cognition over embodiment and the allied assumption that cognition is the exclusive realm of the subject.[5]

But other modes of posthumanist thought do not as readily engage the dualisms of our humanist legacy, and it is these that recapitulate premodern models. Evident in some recent work in robotics, neurophilosophy, and cognitive science, these versions are rightly deemed posthuman, even when they do not explicitly refer to themselves as such, because they counter some of the central characteristics of the distinctly humanist self; they view embodiment as fundamental, as in fact the necessary substrate of human being, consciousness, and selfhood. Focused on a creature's fully embodied existence, these forms of posthumanism typically consider cognitive capacity and agency to be widely distributed phenomena, rather than exclusively localized in an autonomous, conscious, and individuated *mind*, and they assess intelligence in terms of a creature's embedded, networked, and fully imbricated behaviors among manifold social and natural environments.

A ready example of this mode of posthumanism is the work of Rodney Brooks, Director of the MIT Computer Science and Artificial Intelligence Laboratory, whose work with mobile robots in the 1990s revolutionized the field. In the paradigm used by the so-called old AI, mobile robots typically employed a centralized control system, what Brooks calls a "cognition box." In order to navigate their way through a particular space, these systems would first compare information about the local environment gathered by the robot's sensors to a model of that environment preprogrammed into the robot's centralized computer. Then they would figure out, based on the relation between the scanned information and the built-in model, what to tell the actuators in the robot to do. This process involved quite a bit of number crunching and would take some time, so there was always an inelegant (even an "unintelligent") time lag between the sensing and the subsequent moving. The process as a whole, though, was based on the idea that the robot's "intelligence" was situated in its computer "brain," which, especially in early versions of such robots, was housed in a mainframe computer physically separated from the mechanical robot itself.[6]

Brooks's innovation was to dispense with this centralized intelligence system, in essence, to do away with the need for mind conceived of as abstract cognition. As an alternative, he began to build robots that relied on direct sensory-motor loops, on unmediated connections between what the robots sensed and what they did, with no detailed models of the world between them.[7] Brooks built robots from the bottom up, employing relatively simple and autonomous programs, each designed to perform a specific task. The robots were able to act efficiently, even "intelligently," in their environments through *distributed* control systems rather than a centralized plan—that is, through groups of autonomously operating software programs that, functioning in concert, gave rise to complex behaviors that were not themselves programmed into the machines. The intelligence was not *in* the computer brain; rather, it *emerged* through the robots' embodied interaction with their environments.

An early example of such a robot is Genghis, now housed at the National Air and Space Museum in Washington, D.C. Genghis is an insect-like, six-legged robot designed to be able to follow any mammal's path without human intervention. Whereas previous robots designed to navigate space would have to compare whatever they actually encountered in their environment with the model of that environment built into their centralized computer brain and only then determine how to act in the world, Genghis was designed with fifty-one independent, parallel programs, each, Brooks says, no more complex than the software that runs a soda machine.[8] These programs were not centrally integrated (other than minimally, to resolve conflicts); instead, each program interacted with the world on its own to perform a single task based on local and relatively simple computations. When they worked together in a particular environment, however, they enabled Genghis to demonstrate "intelligent" behavior—in this case, following the track of a mammal—without a human controller or a computerized cognition box running the show.

In describing Genghis and the humanoid robots that he has worked on more recently, Brooks alludes to the ways in which his robots engage currently competing models of intelligence and selfhood. Control-box robots manifest what is essentially a reified version of an Enlightenment model: a discrete intelligence responds to and subsequently guides a body's interaction with its environment; agency is localized, centered in the robot's control-box "mind."[9] By contrast, Brooks's bottom-up model is based on an understanding of intelligence as being both fully *embodied* and inextricably *embedded* in local environments. Without a central control box, intelligent behavior emerges as a global effect of simple, systemwide behaviors that are mediated through the world.[10]

Understood with these emphases of *embodiment*, *embeddedness*, and *distributed capacity*, the posthuman need not be confined to its typical realms of artificial intelligence, robotics, and science fiction. Nor need it be exclusively based in the interlacing of human and machine entities, though that certainly is its most common form. One can also see aspects of the posthuman in the feminist epistemology of Elizabeth Grosz, which emphasizes the body's constitutive role in subjectivity; in Donna Haraway's idea of "situated knowledge," which emphasizes the context sensitivity and necessary partiality of knowledge; and in the cognitive science of Francisco Varela, which understands cognition as necessarily and simultaneously embedded and materially situated in the world.[11] But the posthuman selves most pertinent to my purposes are those that emerge from some current research in neuroscience and neurophilosophy, because these imagine selfhood specifically in relation to human biology.

That one can talk at all about brain sciences having anything more or less explicit to say about the self is, of course, a relatively new phenomenon. Until recently, questions related to the contours of selfhood were considered fundamentally philosophical, or perhaps psychophilosophical, in nature, and they were typically addressed by means of introspection and logical analysis. Now, however, partly as a result of developments in neural imaging technologies, brain science has begun to tackle some of these questions head on.[12] What accounts biologically for the existence of consciousness? What gives rise, both evolutionarily and within the individual, to a sense of self, of I-ness? Can agency reasonably be understood as free will?—these questions are now open to empirical analysis.[13]

Precisely because neuroscience could now venture into traditionally philosophical territory, a new discipline, neurophilosophy, emerged in the 1980s to come to terms with what neuroscientific research amounted to philosophically. Neurophilosophy, in other words, is a field of inquiry that approaches topics traditionally considered within the bounds of philosophy (for example, the nature of mind, volition, and the self) from the specific vantage point of neuroscience. Its guiding premise is not simply that neuroscience has something useful to say about these deeply entrenched and knotty philosophical questions but, more strongly, that the best way to make progress on them is to reconsider them in light of neuroscientific research. Patricia Churchland, arguably the founder of the field, has even proposed that it no longer makes sense to pursue epistemology other than in neuroscientific terms.[14]

Though biologically grounded studies of these broad questions are currently quite widespread, it is important to recognize that there is no consensus within either philosophical or scientific communities that neuroscience can ultimately answer them. The skepticism comes from those whom Owen Flanagan calls the "New Mysterians," who argue, for example, that consciousness, because it is by definition subjective and phenomenological, simply cannot be objectively explained, and from functionalists, who do not consider the material substrate of consciousness and cognition to be central to the study of intelligent behavior. Even among those who endorse the usefulness of neuroscientific studies to questions of consciousness and cognition, there is little agreement on whether the widely demonstrated *correlation* between mental and neural events leads or amounts to an *identity* between them; that is, just seeing some physical event on a brain imaging machine at the same time that the subject reports experiencing a mental event does not necessarily mean that the physical event (an implied pattern of neural firing) causes or is identical to the mental event (say, seeing the color red). The two phenomena are clearly correlated but no one is ready to state definitively what the correlation amounts to.[15] And even for those who believe it possible in particular cases, scientific reduction—the explanation of a macrophenomenon in terms of causative physical structures, that is, as an effect of microphenomena—appears to be a long way off and there is no expectation of finding a one-to-one correspondence that explains higher order effects such as perception in terms of the lowest levels of neural activity.[16]

Still, many now think it fully plausible to develop wholly materialist and naturalistic brain-based frameworks for capacities that have in the popular imagination of the past several hundred years traditionally been accorded to a disembodied mind. Robust research in neuroscience is now yielding results that unequivocally demonstrate that the mind's capacities are *materially* made, emerge from widely *distributed* neural networks, and function in fully *embedded* connection with their environments. What is being eroded by contemporary biological studies, therefore, is precisely the model of personhood whose consolidation in the bio-medicine of the early modern period this book studies. If the liberal humanist/ Enlightenment model imagines a self both epistemologically and ontologically separable from the body, a self that wills in a causal vacuum (an unmoved mover) and can therefore freely and autonomously direct its course, and a self that from its inviolable perch within the individual is cut off (and hence free) from its material context, modern neuroscience imagines a self constituted by exactly the opposite characteristics.

Though they disagree on much, there appears to be consensus among both neurophilosophers and philosophical neuroscientists (by which I mean practicing neuroscientists who write about the philosophical implications of their work) that there is simply no basis on which to support a belief in the self as an entity separable either from the body as a whole or from the brain's general capacities. In a way, this is a position not unknown to the Enlightenment, and neu-rophilosophers typically point to Hume's famous observation that he was unable to isolate his self detached from some specific act of perception. "For my part," he wrote, "when I enter most intimately into what I call myself, I always stum-ble on some particular perception or other, of heat or of cold, light or shade, love or hatred, pain or pleasure. I can never catch myself at any time without a per-ception and never can observe anything but the perception."[17] As Flanagan has noted, Hume is not here denying the existence of the self per se but rather the existence of a self all on its own.[18] In other words, whereas it is possible to iso-late and point to parts of one's physical self (to one's thumb, for example) or to the quality of specific experiences one has (as in "this is pain I am feeling"), it is not possible, Hume realized, to point to a *self* outside of its connection to the myriad phenomena of experience.[19]

Modern neuroscience, endorsing Hume's observation, now grounds the results of individual introspection in the findings of empirical research. Evidence gleaned from neural imaging studies and computer modeling of neurological functions suggests that the self, far from being separable and isolated, is a brain-based construct that coordinates an organism's physiological functions and estab-lishes a divide between self and non-self at the deepest and oldest evolutionary levels; one obvious result of such a divide is that an animal does not eat itself when it is hungry. At higher evolutionary levels, the self provides the basis for capacities we more typically associate with selfhood, such as self-representation, self-reflection, planning for the future, and long-term memory. Little is known about the details of how this works, of how the brain generates this sense of I-ness we have, but one of the current ideas is that the self is built from the brain's capacity to *represent to itself* the organism's somatic state and experiences both in the present and over time.[20] For example, at the level of the so-called proto-self, the somatic sensory system and the autonomic nervous system help to create unconscious representational models of the body's physiological condition, including, for example, its heart rate, blood pressure, and glucose level. These models in turn help the organism regulate and coordinate its behavior, helping determine, for example, whether "fight or flight" or "rest and digest" is best suited to its current needs.[21] Whatever the mechanisms of its operation, the important point here is that this most rudimentary, base-level sense of self—an organism's unconscious, psychophysiological self—is neurally constituted.

Demonstrating the neural basis of higher levels of self—what Antonio Dama-sio calls the core self (which is conscious) and the autobiographical self (which also is conscious but involves in addition an extended memory)—is somewhat dicier, but here, too, there is evidence that the very real sense we have of our selves is brain-based and brain-built.[22] Damasio, a cognitive neuroscientist at the University of Iowa, has for decades studied the correlation between brain damage, whether from disease, injury, or congenital defect, and specific neurological deficits associated with emotions, consciousness, and the sense of self. The case histories he writes of them indicate his convictions about the grounding of the self in the body. To take but one example, David (a pseudonym) is a patient who suffered profound damage to his right and left temporal lobes after a severe attack of encephalitis. As a result, he lost nearly all his capacity for memory outside of a one-minute window. He cannot remember the details of his life before the onset of his disease and he cannot retain any currently learned information beyond about 45 seconds. In the immediate present (that is, within the 45–second window) he is fully conscious and functional, but his awareness and sense of self exist only as an unconnected sequence of present moments. He has no extended memory and thus no autobiographical self. Damasio learns much from his study of David and other patients like him—lessons, for example, about the relation between memory and selfhood and about the ability to distinguish *biologically* among the types of capacities we associate with the self. David can speak self-referentially about immediate feelings and desires; he can say, for example, that he is cold or that he wants a cup of coffee, and so, he clearly has some sense of a core self though not of the more elaborate, temporally consistent autobiographical self. But the most general lesson, and certainly the most unequivocal for Damasio, is that the damage to David's *self* results specifically from damage to his *brain*. To emphasize the point, Damasio compares David's condition to that of another patient, H. M., who, like David, cannot learn new facts. But unlike David, H. M. *does* remember his past. What explains their differing capacities is that whereas both David and H. M. suffered damage to the hippocampus, only David has additional lesions in the cortices of the rest of his temporal lobes.[23]

A myriad such studies correlate deficits in aspects of one's self—memory, body image, and so forth—with specific kinds of brain damage. What they cumulatively suggest is that the self is a brain-based construct at all levels and cannot be understood as separate from the process of the brain's activity. The self, then, is the cognitive effect of a fully embodied process. Patricia Churchland has nicely assessed the implication of this commitment to embodiment: from the evidence of human biology, it is now possible to assert that there is no homuncular self, no "extra-neural 'mini-me'" inside one's head that shines a light on the physical activity of the brain and transforms it into the mental world of consciousness.[24]

The self as an effect of embodiment accords with research that demonstrates more generally the materiality of the mind. Neuroscience frees itself most clearly from the legacy of substance dualism—the idea that mind is made up of something essentially other than and different from matter—in the many studies that point to a correlation and, in some instances, even a relationship of clear dependence between mental capacities and brain anatomy and activity. Among the oldest of these are the so-called split-brain studies of the 1960s, in which experiments were performed with patients who had had severed the nerve network that connects the right and left cerebral hemispheres of the brain as a last-ditch treatment for certain types of epilepsy that were not susceptible to drug therapies. In these postoperative experiments researchers found that each hemisphere was able to function separately under certain circumstances, providing independent, and disparate, conscious experiences to the patients. Flanagan describes one of the many experiments:

> If [the words] *key* and *ring* are flashed on the left and right sides of the visual field respectively [and thus processed, respectively, by the right and left hemispheres], and the person is told to retrieve what she saw from a group of objects behind a screen, her two hands will work independently. The right hand will reject the key and settle on the ring; the left hand will do the opposite.[25]

Patricia Churchland describes another experiment, set up differently but yielding the same results:

> A picture of a snowy scene is flashed to the right hemisphere, and a picture of a chicken's claw is flashed to the left. An array of pictures is placed before the subject, who is to select, with each hand, the picture that best matches the flashed picture. In this set-up, the split-brain subject does this: his left hand (controlled by the right hemisphere) points to a shovel to go with the snowy scene, and the right hand (controlled by the left hemisphere) selects a chicken's head to go with the chicken's claw.[26]

These and other experiments performed on split-brain patients provided a lot of information about the brain's functional organization (for example, that the left and right cerebral hemispheres are associated with opposite sides of the body) but they also provided tantalizing clues about the material basis of consciousness: the unity of the consciousness we normally experience seems to depend on the *anatomical* unity of the brain itself.[27]

The reliance of the mental on the physical is also shown in the many correspondences discovered between all manner of neuropsychological deficits and damage to specific regions of the brain, of which Damasio's patient David is one case. The examples here are numerous: lesions in the association cortex of the right hemisphere correlate with an inability to recognize faces; damage to the right parietal lobe is affiliated with a condition known as hemineglect, in which a person is aware of only the left side of his visual field and thus, for example, will shave only the left side of his face or, when asked to copy a picture presented to him, will draw only its left side; and damage to the parietal cortex of the right hemisphere is associated with limb denial, a condition in which a patient denies that her left arm or leg actually is her own and so might, for example, attempt to toss it out of a hospital bed. (Significantly, this condition occurs only with damage to the right hemisphere; patients whose left parietal cortex is compromised experience no such abnormality vis-à-vis their right limbs).[28]

These findings demonstrate how large-scale mental capacities like bodily self-representation and coherent vision depend on correspondingly large-scale anatomical features of the brain. Other research proposes these correspondences at the neural level as well; the most widely known among these is perhaps Gerald Edelman's theory of neural Darwinism, which proposes a theory of consciousness based on the premise that the general principles of Darwinian natural selection, along with elaborate systems of feedback loops, apply in the development of the massively complex neural connections that our conscious brains possess.[29] Together, this wide-ranging work in brain science makes untenable the notion of a self, of mind, of consciousness, as something separable from matter and existing a priori in human nature.

The embodied self proposed by modern neuroscience, constructed not by a homuncular mini-me but rather by the brain's interactions with the rest of the body and the environment, is a posthuman model, not in the common sense of melding human and machine but in the more specific sense of being materially constructed and located, networked into context, and fully functional without a centralized and separable leader. This refiguration of the posthuman to include but not be restricted by the human-machine interface is neatly typified in the work of Andy Clark, a philosopher of mind and cognitive scientist at Indiana University. As he suggests by the title of his recent book, *Natural-Born Cyborgs*,

Clark believes that the interlacing of humans and the intelligent technologies that are available to us today and that will become increasingly available in the future (cochlear and retinal implants, various forms of telepresence, wearable computers, among others) do not constitute a revolutionary development in the evolution of either the human species or our culture. Rather, he argues, our interaction with these technologies and "cognitive props" perpetuates what has always been true, and distinctly true, about human beings—that the astonishingly plastic human mind is continuously able to construct *and be constructed by* "an empowering web of culture, education, technology, and artifacts."[30] He maintains that the conception of the mind or self as being isolated in what he calls the "skin-bag" of our skulls has always been an illusion; the cognitive system and the self it supports actually comprise and are distributed among mind, body, and world.

Clark makes his argument by considering our current and future interactions with highly advanced information technologies, but the point is easily recognized in one of his most mundane examples in which he asks us to consider our use of a wristwatch. If someone on the street asks you if you know the time, typically (assuming you are wearing a watch), you say "Yes, I do" *before*, if only a second before, actually looking at your watch. You would never respond the same way to a query about a word you do not know, even if you had a dictionary close by. The point, Clark says, is that the ubiquitous and easily accessible wristwatch, unlike the more cumbersome dictionary, has in a sense merged with our sense of what constitutes our self:

> The ease with which we accept talk of the watch-bearer as one who actually knows—rather than one who can easily find out—the time is suggestive. For the line between that which is *easily and readily accessible* and that which should be counted as *part of the knowledge base* of an active intelligent system is slim and unstable indeed. It is so slim and unstable, in fact, that it sometimes makes both social and scientific sense to think of your individual knowledge as quite simply whatever body of information and understanding is at your fingertips. . . . According to one diagnosis, then, you are telling the literal truth when you answer "yes" to the innocent-sounding question "Do you know the time?" For you *do* know the time. It is just that the "you" that knows the time is no longer the bare biological organism but the hybrid biotechnological system that now includes the wristwatch as a proper part.[31]

One could contest the adequacy of the example but the argument remains appealing: it is only a matter of convention to think of a self as bounded in the biological borders of an organism; it would be more accurate, Clark argues, to think of that organism as contiguous with its context, rather than somehow occupying a particular place *in* it. This is what he means, I think, by what he calls the "soft self":

> There is *no self*, if by self we mean some central cognitive essence that makes me who and what I am. In its place there is just the "soft self": a rough-and-tumble, control-sharing coalition of processes—some neural, some bodily, some technological—and an ongoing drive to tell a story, to paint a picture in which "I" am the central player. . . . The notion of a real, central, wafer-thin self is a profound mistake. It is a mistake that blinds us to our real nature and leads us to radically undervalue and misconceive the roles of context, culture, environment, and technology in the *constitution* of individual human persons. To face up to our true nature (soft selves, distributed decentralized coalitions) is to recognize the inextricable intimacy of self, mind, world.[32]

Clark recognizes, as do others writing about our already or always posthuman nature, that this model of the human being, though perhaps old hat in certain academic departments, goes against the grain of contemporary western culture. Flanagan's recent book, *The Problem of the Soul*, is essentially a response to this very concern. He argues unequivocally that there is no scientific basis for the understanding of the human that pervades our society but he assures us that we need not be frightened by what modern brain science suggests, that even if we give up (as we must) the earmarks of the humanist image (nonphysical minds and immutable selves, for example), we can still hold on to the idea of a person as "a conscious social animal that deliberates, reasons, and chooses, that is possessed of an evolving or continuous—but not permanent or immutable—identity, and that seeks to live morally and meaningfully."[33]

Hayles, too, realizes that the posthuman strikes some as alarming, and she herself speaks with alarm about some versions of it, particularly those that perpetuate the humanist legacy of disembodied minds and separable selves. But the point I want to make is that the features of the posthuman that I am attending to are alarming *only* from the perspective of the liberal humanist subject, because the posthuman sacrifices the fundamental premises of the humanist self—(the façade of) autonomy, self-directedness, and the hegemony of mind over matter. Of course, humanism and posthumanism are equally historical constructs, produced in the contexts of the particular exigencies and opportunities of their periods. But the posthuman begins to look more normative (and thus less alarming), the humanist itself more aberrant, when the posthuman is placed beside the premodern for comparison. I want to propose that, rather than being radically new, these recurrent features of the posthuman recapitulate in a different register distinctive aspects of the premodern Galenic person.

■  Galen of Pergamon was a second-century medical man, surgeon to gladiators and physician to Emperor Marcus Aurelius in Rome. Over the course of decades of practice, observation, and experiment, Galen wrote on anatomy, physiology, pharmacology, and on the causes as well as the treatment of disease. He wrote voluminously, both original works and commentaries on his philosophical and medical predecessors (the modern Greek edition of his works, edited in the nineteenth century, comprises twenty-two volumes). Drawing on the medical wisdom of Hippocrates and his successors, steeped in the philosophies of Plato and Aristotle, Galen composed his works in constant and energetic debate with both earlier medical authorities and with contemporary rival schools of thought. He crystallized the main elements of Greek medicine, amplified them and drew syncretically from their many sources, and it was his numerous writings—themselves amplified and systematized over the centuries—that grounded the dominant mode of medical theory and practice in the West for nearly a millennium and a half.

My intent here is neither to offer a synoptic introduction to Galen's many works nor to rehearse the story of Galenism's rise and eventual decline.[34] Rather, I want briefly to set out those aspects of Galenic physiology that suggest most clearly the pattern of the Galenic person.[35] Although there is in Galenic vocabulary no word for self—even less a trace of what a modern might mean by that freighted term—it is nonetheless possible to limn the parameters of Galenic personhood and to consider what understanding of the human being underwrites Galen's thinking about the functioning of the human body. I will argue that in ways quietly evocative of the posthuman, the Galenic person is embedded in the world, grounded in the body, and conceptualized as a unity in the distributed functioning of the psychosomatic system. Whatever the ineluctable differences between Galenic and posthuman bio-medicine, the areas of affinity are real and they appear even more pronounced by contrast with the humanist self that superceded the one and is now in turn being dismantled by the other. My point in noting these affinities is not to propose that the premodern in any way *anticipates* the posthuman; it is rather to suggest some level of continuity in the western tradition that is broken most starkly for only a few hundred years. [36]

■ That the Galenic person is wholly and inextricably embedded in the world is perhaps most clearly evident in the pervasive reach of the theory of the four qualities that Galen inherited from his philosophical and medical predecessors. This theory held that all things are characterized by four mutually interacting qualities: warm and cold, moist and dry, and the particular interaction and operation of these qualities, Galen said, accounted for "the genesis and destruction of all things that come into and pass out of being."[37] These qualities were, or were associated with, the four basic elements of matter—earth, water, air, and fire—which mixed in different proportions in every natural thing. Galen considered this material mixing to be the universally present ground of all alteration, growth, and decay and the foundation of health and disease. So encompassing was the explanatory reach of this idea that anything in nature could be understood according to its own particular mixture of these qualities. Thus, the elements themselves and all material things, but also the seasons, the stages of life, nations, the sexes—each had its particular mixture of warm and cold, moist and dry.

In the living body, the qualities and elements were expressed as the humors, also four in number: blood, phlegm, yellow bile, and black bile. Galen theorized about the exact relation of the humors to their grounding qualities, but generally he considered the humors to be those substances in which the various mixtures of the primary qualities were manifest in the body. Each humor was characterized by some mixture of the qualities: black bile, analogous to earth, was cold and dry; phlegm, analogous to water, was cold and moist; yellow bile, like fire, was warm and dry; blood, the air-like element, was warm and moist. Galen took pains to stress that the qualities of any substance were not absolutes but relative, either within or across kinds. For example, phlegm is cold and moist not absolutely and in itself, but in relation, say, to blood, which is warm and moist. This was important for a physician to understand because the qualities combined in varying proportions in different parts of the living body to give every part a particular humoral mixture relative to every other part. Furthermore, as a person was constituted by his or her parts, every individual, depending on age, sex, occupation, diet, living condition, and particular material makeup, had a particular mixture or balance, a *krasis* or temperament, that was uniquely proper to him or her. Health therefore ensued in individuals when the humors were mixed proportionately according to each person's particular temperament; disease resulted from an imbalance, from any humor growing excessive, deficient, or putrefying in the body.

Because the qualities occur universally, in "nature, disease, time of life, season of the year, locality, [and] occupation" (*NF*, 193), humoral theory, which is based on the mixing of those qualities, enmeshes every aspect of every person in every circumstance. Medicine therefore had to heed the full range of an individual's situation, her or his age, diet, geographical location, the season of the year, because all these aspects conditioned and were conditioned by the different mixings of the qualities.

Diet, for example, was an obvious medical issue because the various mixtures that constitute different foods materially affect the body within which they are digested and transformed into the body's substances. Galen ridiculed those who believed that the different humors were actually present *in* the foods ingested rather than produced by the body in the process of digestion. For this reason, it was particularly important to understand an individual's temperament, because a person's relative mixture of warm, cold, moist, and dry, which itself depended on age, location, sex, season of the year, and so on, determined how that food would be digested and therefore what humors would be produced:

> Those articles of food which are by nature warmer are more productive of bile, and those which are colder produce more phlegm. Similarly of the periods of life, those which are naturally warmer tend more to bile, and the colder more to phlegm. Of occupations also, localities and seasons, and above all, of natures themselves, the colder are more phlegmatic, and the warmer more bilious. Also cold diseases result from phlegm, and warmer ones from yellow bile. . . . [E]very part functions in its own special way because of the manner in which the four qualities are compounded. (*NF*, 183, 185)

Foods have their own inherent mixtures, but because their function in a body depends on the mixture of the four qualities in that particular body, not all foods are appropriate for all people, or even for the same person through all periods of life. Thus, for example, honey, which is naturally warm, can become dangerously warm and bilious in people who are already warm because of, say, the season or their age:

> [H]oney is therefore bad in bilious diseases but good in old age; . . . it is harmful for those who are naturally bilious, and serviceable for those who are phlegmatic. In a word, in bodies which are warm either through nature, disease, time of life, season

of the year, locality, or occupation, honey is productive of bile, whereas in opposite circumstances it produces blood. (*NF*, 193)

Climate, season, location, lifestyle, diet, sex—all these factors mattered in establishing and maintaining proper *krasis* because all were characterized by the same mixing of the four foundational qualities.

Given the ubiquity of the qualities, in people's bodies as well as in the texture of the world, it was not possible in the Galenic economy to consider a person as an inviolable entity *in* the world, as one who, separate in essence, interacted with the world as something external to it. Rather, a person was fully and materially *embedded* in the world, constituted by the same qualities that made up the world. A person was not so much an autonomous entity in the world as *a particular point in a network of relations* that constituted every aspect of the world.

Timothy Reiss, who has considered this understanding of human being across the ancient and medieval West, characterizes it thus: "Being was indivisible from a total ecosystem experienced . . . as a universe of sympathies among [manifold] surroundings. . . . [T]he tie between human constitution and character, nutrition, physical condition, climate, geographic place, planets and zodiac was axiomatic."[38] These aspects of existence, Reiss explains, were not conceived of as *essentially* separate from the person; they were, rather, the "existential spheres to which the person enlaced in them was in a reactive relation."[39] Reiss calls this reactive enlacing "passibility," which he defines as "experiences of being whose common denominator was a sense of being *embedded in* and acted on by these circles—including the material and immediate biological, familial and social ambiences, as well as the soul's . . . cosmic, spiritual and divine life."[40]

It is Reiss's argument that this notion of the "passible *selfe*," pervades ancient philosophical, medical, and political culture and remains fairly constant, although with increasingly notable dissonance, up to the sixteenth and seventeenth centuries, when the modern myth of the inviolable, essential, disembodied self is fully formulated. This myth was literally inconceivable for Galen because the theory of qualities made seamless the joint between the human and the natural world. Human being was understood as an aspect of a network—not in precisely the same way that Andy Clark conceives of human nature as cyborgian but certainly closer to Clark's sense of a person's proper boundaries beyond the skin-bag of the skull than to the Cartesian sense of an "I" that exists as an isolated, immaterial thinking thing.

If human being is thus understood as embedded, as fully pervious to and consisting of context, it is also understood, medically at least, as fully embodied. Galenic physiology (like much of Greek medicine) makes no clear-cut, ontological distinctions among what we would call the physical, the mental, and the affective aspects of human being. Considered medically, these aspects were all in some sense corporeal and were therefore susceptible to medicine's material intervention. The complex status and physiological role of the psyche (usually translated as "soul") is a case in point.[41] Against the Stoic account of a unitary psyche, Galen preferred Plato's idea of the tripartite psyche comprising the *rational*, which was responsible for sensation, voluntary motion, imagination, memory, and thought; the *vital*, responsible for innate heat and for states of passion; and the *desiderative*, responsible for growth, nutrition, and reproduction. And, again like Plato, he assigned to each soul a seat in the body—the rational resided in the brain, the vital or spirited in the heart, and the desiderative in the liver. But this arrangement of the psyche being "seated" in various organs raises the question of correlation; what does it mean that the rational psyche is *seated* in the brain or that the desiderative psyche is *seated* in the liver? What is the relation of rational soul to brain, of the mental capacity for memory, for example, to the physical structure of the brain? How is psyche related to soma?[42]

Galen generally tended to avow ignorance about the issue; he was not at any rate willing to accede to the Platonists' view that psyche, even the rational psyche, was an a priori entity implanted in the body at birth and thus, in essence, both immaterial and immortal. In *On the Formation of Foetuses*, he wrote: "I made no attempt to assert anything regarding the soul's substance in any of my work. For I was unable to find out by means of linear demonstrations whether it was completely incorporeal, or if some part of it was corporeal, or whether it was completely eternal, or if it was corruptible."[43]

Galen actually thought that such agnosticism was the appropriate stance for a physician to take because even though philosophy and medicine tended to be in complete agreement, a physician needed to speak in terms appropriate to clinical intervention.[44] He addresses the question of the relation of psyche to soma from a different angle in *On the Doctrines of Plato and Hippocrates* but arrives at the same position: "it makes no difference," he says, "whether the liver is called the source of the veins, or of the appetitive soul, but it is more appropriate for a physician to present his teaching in terms of bodily organs, a philosopher in terms of powers of the soul."[45] Whatever his agnosticism about the soul's actual substance, then, Galen considered it both useful and proper for a physician to speak of the soul as materially based and thus as susceptible to material (that is, medical) intervention. As a physician, even a philosophically inclined one, Galen felt it proper to speak functionally rather than ontologically.

Despite his general reluctance to assert a definitive conclusion, Galen did in several works speak directly and pointedly to the question. For example, in *On the Soul's Dependence on the Body*, a small treatise in which he tries to show the essential agreement among Hippocrates, Plato, and Aristotle on the question of the relation of psyche to soma, Galen argues fairly clearly for the corporeality of the soul, that it is bodily and cannot exist without the body, because this is the only way convincingly to explain the myriad psychic changes that are subsequent to bodily harm.

Why does one behave drunkenly after having too much to drink? Why does one become forgetful or delirious after certain drugs are administered or when certain humors accumulate in the body? And why does excessive heat or cold in the body result in death, a condition that all would agree constitutes if not the extinction of the psyche, at least its separation from the body? The only way to explain these changes in psychic state—in behavior, perception, memory, even life status, which are all expressions of psyche—is to assume that psyche is *in some way* grounded in soma.

Galen asks: when people see things that are not present or hear things that no one has said, does that not indicate not just a loss of faculties that the soul innately possesses but the presence of some opposite faculty, that is, the faculty to sense what does not exist? So, he reasons: "Such a consideration may in itself cast doubt on the non-bodily nature of the soul as a whole. For if the soul were not some quality, form, affection, or faculty of the body, how could it actually acquire a nature opposite to its own, just by communion with the body?"[46]

It is important to recognize that Galen is referring here to the soul as a whole and not just to its spirited and desiderative parts. All the soul's capacities, for reason and memory and sentience as much as for anger and hunger and sexual appetite, are faculties fully dependent on the body's material mixture. As he clearly states: "the faculties of the soul depend on the mixtures of the body—and not just the faculties within the spirited and desiderative parts of the soul, but those in the rational part too."[47] Galen is claiming here that the soul's capacities of reasoning and remembering, no less than of desiring and repelling, are material processes, or, at the least, that they are materially dependent.

This idea forms the basis of Galen's materialist psychology, which itself defines Galen's sense of embodied being: if a person's character traits—whether abstemious

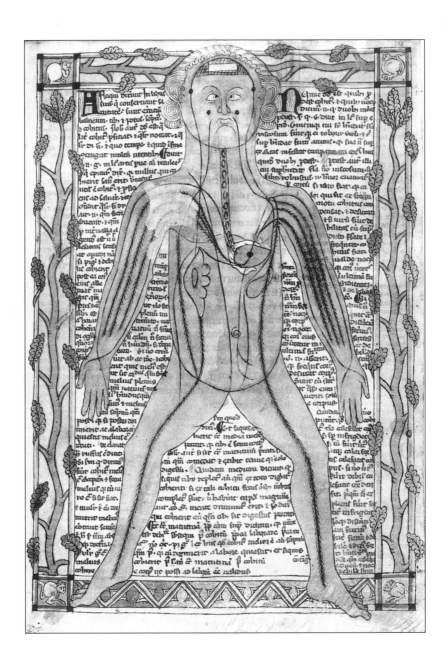

*Plate 1. From Ashmole Manuscript 399; thirteenth-century illustration, depicting the flow of psychic pneuma to the organs and extremities. Reproduced by permission of the Bodleian Library.*

or indulgent, brave or cowardly, shrewd or foolish—are an expression of their psychic function, and if psyche depends on the material mixture of the body, it follows that personhood, at least in so far as it entails one's character, must be understood as being embodied. The body is thus the basis not only of *what* a person materially is but of *who* and *how* a person is in the world.

Galen's commitment to embodied being does not, however, lead to a strict biological determinism, to the sense that the body's particular configuration determines exclusively the status of the whole organism. With Aristotle and the Hippocratics before him, Galen built a teleological physiology that assumed that all the parts of the living animal were created by a wise and provident Nature with the purpose of promoting the overall well-being of the whole. In part, Galen's commitment to teleology explains his ambivalence about the substance of the soul. As much as he asserts in one treatise that the soul follows from the mixtures of the body, he elsewhere holds that the body follows the dictates of the soul; the *pneuma*, for example, is frequently described as the "first instrument" of the psyche, the material means by which the psyche's acts are carried out (see plate 1).[48] For a physician, just as the status of the substance or mortality of the soul is ultimately irrelevant, so, too, is the question of the causal order of body and soul; on a practical, clinical level, what mattered was not determining the priority of one of the elements (whether soul follows from body or body from soul), but *the inextricable interrelation between them in the living being*. In clinical practice, psychophysiology worked in both directions: a physician might recommend a change in diet to relieve a psychic disease just as, in other circumstances, he might find that a physical disease is affected by mental activity. Thus Galen writes that "it is possible for mental activity itself to be the cause of health or illness. . . . There are many who do not die because of the pernicious nature of their illness but because of the poor state of their mind and reason."[49]

In his treatise *On the Passions and Errors of the Soul*, Galen recommends education and moral counseling as the best means of treating any unhealthy inclination of the soul, for greed, say, or for anger. Yet *On the Soul's Dependence on the Body* asserts that psychic life, "the habits of the soul," are affected, even determined, by a person's bodily mixture. This ambivalence in Galen's writings is an effect of his desire to devise a full range of viable therapeutics. But it also suggests an ontology of the organism in which, practically speaking, psyche and soma are mutually determining, each in some regard, or at some time, potentially dependent on the other, interacting in a system of relations that does not permit a one-way traffic from cause to effect; in the practice of medicine, soma and psyche are each both cause and effect of the other. If this economy saves Galen from an unmitigated biological determinism, it also points to his dual commitment—to a soul that is embodied and a body that is vital in all its parts.

Galen's adherence to the tripartite model of the psyche also points to the last of the three areas of overlap I want to mention, and that is the idea that high-level capacity (like perception) is not localized in a single control center but distributed throughout the body's psychosomatic system. The rational part of the soul, responsible for what we would call cognitive faculties, such as sentience, voluntary motion, reason, and memory, was, for Galen, the *hegemonikon*, or the ruling part of the soul, and he performed numerous experiments to demonstrate that the hegemonikon was seated in the brain and not in the heart, as Aristotle had maintained.[50] However, although the rational soul was brain-based, the brain did not have a monopoly on cognition or perception. In Galenic physiology, the organs of the body are endowed with faculties that enable them to *perceive* their needs. What Galen called the four natural faculties—attractive, retentive, alterative, and expulsive—enable the organs to carry out their functions: to attract whatever is necessary to them, to retain it for as long as they need, to transform it to a substance appropriate to their needs, and then to expel whatever is left over. This system of faculties accounts among other things for the separation of bile from blood in the liver, the expulsion of urine from the bladder, and the entire process of digestion: the stomach attracts food, retains is as long as is necessary to transform it to chyle, which constitutes the basis of the body's nourishment, and then expels the waste products from its cavity.

In order for the system to work, however, the parts have to *know* what is necessary to them and what is not; they have somehow to know what to attract and what to expel. Though he explains that the power of perception is not innate to the parts but comes from the nerves carrying psychic pneuma to them (*UP*, 209), Galen's descriptions of how the natural faculties work typically personify the parts, treating them as if they were autonomous agents and endowing them with both the appetites and the cognitive capacities that we, in a more humanist vein, might more readily ascribe to a supervenient self than to any particular organ in the body. The stomach, Galen says, "craves" nourishment and "devours" whatever it finds useful until it is thoroughly "satisfied" (*UP*, 211). It furthermore knows both what to crave and when because it has been granted the "power of perception of what is lacking," and so it has "the ability to feel a lack which arouses the animal and stimulates it to seek food" (*UP*, 208). In Galen's description, it is the stomach that hungers, that craves food, and not the animal as a whole. The animal exists, in fact, not as an a priori center of volition but as the object of an agency that is expressed originally in an organ.

A similar distribution of capacities applies to the many loci of desire. Though the desiderative psyche has its seat in the liver, it is not the liver alone (or even the body more generally, as opposed to mind) that desires, for Galen says that the rational soul, too, desires; "that part of the soul which we call the rational is desiderative in the broad sense of that term: it desires truth, knowledge, learning, understanding, and recollection—in short, all the goods" (*UP*, 152). Similarly, the spirited or vital psyche desires "freedom, victory, power, authority, reputation, and honor," and the desiderative psyche desires "sexual pleasure . . . and the enjoyment of all kinds of food and drink" (ibid.). So, it is not possible to think of the mind's cognition on the one hand and the body's appetites on the other, as we commonly might. Galen's scheme is more integrated than that; the desire for sex or food or honor is as much a psychic (or ensouled) function as is the desire for truth. Desire is not localized in any one part of the body because it is a function of an embodied psyche that pervades the organism as a whole.

So, too, with the passions, which, though seated in the heart, seem to be experienced by all the parts of the body: There must, Galen asserts,

> exist in almost all parts of the animal a certain inclination towards, or, so to speak, an appetite for their own special quality, and an aversion to, or, as it were, a hatred of the foreign quality. And it is natural that when they feel an inclination they should attract, and that when they feel aversion they should expel. (*NF*, 247–49)

The organs themselves experience affect; they are inclined toward what is familiar and hate what is foreign to them; they act themselves as a person might in love or anger.

From a humanist perspective, this is a rather uncomfortable notion, this idea that perception and desire and affect are not localized in a unified mind, that what to us are generally attributes of a *person*, such as desire and perception, are possessed instead by material *parts* such as stomachs or livers.[51] And you can see this discomfort at work as Galen scholars consider his physiological system. R. J. Hankinson asks about Galen's conflation of attraction (a material process of bodies) and desire (an affective process of the self). The two, he points out, are not the same thing, especially if we think of desire as a conscious act. Hankinson sees Galen caught in a logical fallacy. Using the liver as his example, he paraphrases Galen's argument: my liver tries to get food, I try to get food; hence

I (qua my desire for nutrition) am my liver.[52] Hankinson tries to reason Galen out of his difficulty but the point, I think, is that it is a difficulty *only from a humanist perspective*, one that thinks of the self only as consciousness localized in a disembodied mind rather than as a collection of distributed, embodied components.

Hankinson is similarly troubled by the idea of the tripartite soul, and for similar reasons. He notes that in the Stoic account of the unitary soul, "the identity of the agent is never in doubt," whereas in accounts of psychic conflict that are based in the tripartite soul, "one is tempted . . . to ask just *who* it is within whom the warring factions contend."[53] How, he wonders, can "the different bits . . . function as a coherent whole" so that "it can seem to the individuals that they *are* individuals, and not collections." But the question assumes that the self *is* unitary and localized, that it is a bounded thing and not enacted in a distributed process. Why *cannot* the "who" be a collection as it is for the posthuman; Katherine Hayles attests: "the posthuman subject is an amalgam, a collection of heterogeneous components."[54] Think of Galen as you listen to Katherine Hayles describe her experience of being a posthuman person: "I now find myself saying things like, 'Well, my sleep agent wants to rest, but my food agent says I should go to the store.' Each person who thinks this way begins to envision herself or himself as a posthuman collectivity, an 'I' transformed into the 'we' of autonomous agents operating together to make a self."[55]

It must be said that Galen's belief in a teleological physiology does distance him from the posthuman, indeed from all secular conceptions of human being. Aside from the many differences in anatomical and physiological detail (our blood circulates, for example, and it does not turn into semen), Galen's teleology arguably constitutes the most fundamental divide between his and the posthuman vision because teleology is premised on a purposiveness in nature that strictly secular viewpoints typically deride. The underwriting premise of Galen's central treatises on anatomy and physiology, *On the Usefulness of the Parts* and *On the Natural Faculties*, is precisely a demonstration of this teleology. Nature, working with what Galen calls "creative ingenuity and forethought" (*UP*, 185), has shaped all the parts of the body and endowed them with capacities in the best possible way to function together for the sake of the whole organism. Each part is conceived of as constituting and functioning on behalf of an organic, vital whole. Conceptually, then, the whole, the that-for-whose-sake, precedes the parts and their faculties. In this regard, Galen's understanding is worlds away from the one underlying, say, Brooks's robot Genghis, whose parts function in near autonomy and whose purposiveness emerges from its action in the world. But practically, in the functioning of the lived body, the powers of perception, the faculties of desire, of attraction and repulsion, are for Galen fully distributed in the organism and are not localizable in anything to be conceived of as a separable, independent self.

For Galen, anything that we would term the self is a distributed entity, a pattern that arises from the functioning in concert of the body's manifold parts. The tripartite psyche is a collection, and the psychic faculties that the parts of the body possess demonstrate their coherence through interactive functioning. The rational soul may be the ruling part of the soul but it is not for that reason the exclusive locus of cognition broadly conceived any more than it is the single locus of personhood. It is the humanist perspective that makes the stomach's perception of hunger seem bizarre, because perception is something it attributes to *mind*, or more colloquially to a self that is coterminus with mind. But it should not seem bizarre from the Galenic perspective in which, despite the teleology, there is no supervening self that oversees the functioning of the organism.

Discussing this tendency to grant not only faculties but perception to body parts, the editors of an influential collection of essays, *The Body in Parts*, view the somatic subjectification evident in numerous early modern texts as decidedly "eery," and it seems eery to the editors precisely for the reasons that make Hankinson uncomfortable—it suggests that an organism is a collection of autonomous parts, rather than a natural and naturally coherent individual.[56] But I think the editors have got the eeriness precisely wrong; perhaps from the humanist position from which they (unwittingly) write, Galenic models *are* eery but from the arc that stretches from Galen to Hayles, from a perspective that embraces the premodern and the posthuman, the eeriness resides in the model in the middle. For Galen, as for Hayles (as, for that matter, for Brooks and Damasio and Clark as well), anything that can reasonably be called the self is a group effort, manifest in the functioning together of the parts of a distributed system. There is for the premodern as for the posthuman no necessary sense of a person that precedes or supervenes the parts. The psyche, the self, the mind, all are or arise from or are in some way implicated in matter. In this sense, these thinkers, both premodern and posthuman, share something with Aristotle, for whom *psyche* meant the kind of organization and functioning that certain pieces of matter have, not a thing in itself, let alone a thing separate from matter, but rather the functional organization of matter endowed with life.[57]

If I am right about this—that in some ways at least, for all its emphasis on the technoscientific modifications of what it means to be human, the posthuman replicates and returns us to certain premodern assumptions about personhood—then the humanist self, that disembodied, vacuum-sealed center of cognition and volition, that self which some hold dear and others dearly endeavor to deride, may perhaps be repositioned from its place of faltering authority to one of anomalous outsider to the western tradition. Perhaps, then, the material in the middle, the early modern bio-medicine this book will study, can tell us something about our own wrestling with the seemingly eery newness of the bodies and selves that constitute our increasingly posthuman culture, namely, that the self notoriously dismantled in the manifold discourses of postmodernity is not only a (mere) construct of the early modern world but also one that neglected something that seems to have been understood long ago, something that is being recapitulated now—the groundedness of being in the particulate workings of a body networked in the world.

ANCIENT REVISIONS

## 2 / Subjectified Parts and Supervenient Selves:

### Rewriting Galenism in Crooke's
# Microcosmographia

THE GALENIC REVIVAL OF THE SIXTEENTH CEN-
tury was made possible and in large measure was constituted by the
nearly six hundred new editions and translations of Galen's works by
humanist scholars in Western Europe.[1] Because, like so much of Greek
learning, only a few of Galen's works had been translated into Latin before the
fall of the Roman Empire, Galenism flourished in the Arabic East much more
than in the Latin West, and it was only after the editions, compilations, and commentaries of the great medieval Jewish and Muslim scholars of philosophy and
medicine became available in Latin in the twelfth century that Galen reemerged
in the West.[2] The medieval Galenism that came to dominate the newly established universities of Western Europe during and after the twelfth century was
thus grounded in Galen as he was understood and systematized by Arabic philosophy and medicine.[3] When Christian humanist scholars gained access to newly
available manuscripts of Galen's works in the sixteenth century, therefore, their
announced intent was to purge the Galenic corpus of what they considered to
be its many medieval and "pagan" corruptions. As one of the leading humanists of Ferrara wrote, earlier editions of Galen had "made medicine to be not
only polluted, uncultured and punic and barbarous . . . but [they] also maimed
and in many parts mutilated" the texts.[4] According to a typical argument of writers conscious of creating a renaissance of classical learning, medicine would now
be able to progress because the knowledge of the ancients had been at last redis-
covered and brought back to its pristine integrity.

In England, Thomas Linacre (c.1460–1524) and John Caius (1510–1573) contrib-
uted a few editions to this effort to retrieve the "original" Galen and make him

available to the world of Latin learning.[5] But the medical renaissance in England came about less through the original work of humanist philological scholars who published in Latin and more through the myriad vernacular medical texts that sought to consolidate bio-medical knowledge and reconcile the purified authority of the ancients with the new discoveries being culled from the anatomy theaters of Renaissance Europe.[6] These vernacular texts based on Galenic learning and comprising anatomies, surgical treatises, and books of practical physic wrought significant changes on the nearly 1,500-year-old bio-medical system they inherited. In part, these changes came from incorporating the factual details of the new anatomy, although, as we shall see, even some of these were open to contest, but more profoundly, if more subtly, the changes also had to do with the notion of personhood these texts limned. In its renditions of embodied being, distributed agency, and contextual embeddedness, the Galenic person, I have argued, has more in common with contemporary notions of the posthuman than it does with the conditions of subjectivity starting to trouble the texts of early modern culture. Much of the vernacular bio-medical literature of sixteenth- and early seventeenth-century England perpetuates the fundamental components of Galenic anatomy and physiology but, even as it does so, it insistently rewrites their workings to support a notion of subjectivity more nearly aligned with masculinist and humanist ideals. Focusing on the rhetorical maneuvers and specific tropings of Helkiah Crooke's magisterial *Microcosmographia: A Description of the Body of Man*, this chapter describes how what has come to be called the liberal humanist subject—supervenient, disembodied, and distinctly masculine— emerges within a physiological system that does not logically require (and would, in fact, logically eschew) such a notion of the self.[7]

■ Crooke begins his enormous English compilation of continental anatomy with a long justification of his endeavor. Although Thomas Vicary and John Banister had published relatively brief, synoptic anatomies in English (in 1548 and 1578, respectively), no one had previously attempted a project approaching the scope of Crooke's, which amounts to over 1,000 small-print folio pages and would have been longer still, Crooke says, "had not the bulke of the volume growne too great, and so too chargeable to the Printer."[8] Crooke's fairly conventional reasons for committing himself to such a daunting enterprise are revealing, precisely because they are routine, not only about the state of anatomy and competitive medicine at the time but also about the contemporary configuration of anatomy's relation to the self.

ΜΙΚΡΟΚΟΣΜΟΓΡΑΦΙΑ:

A

# DESCRIPTION
of the Body of Man.

TOGETHER
VVITH THE CONTROVERSIES
THERETO BELONGING.

*Collected and Translated out of all the Best Authors of Anatomy,
Especially out of* Gasper Bauhinus *and* Andreas Laurentius.

By HELKIAH CROOKE Doctor in Physicke.

—————————*Etiam Parnassia Laurus
Parua, sub ingenti matris se subijcit vmbra.*

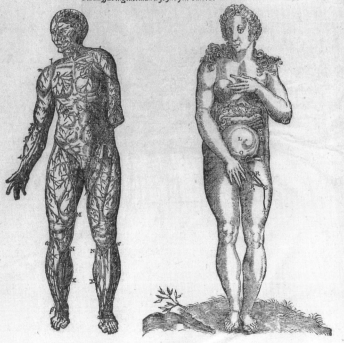

LONDON,
Printed by William Iaggard dwelling in Barbican, and are there to be sold, 1615.

*Plate 2. Title page of Helkiah Crooke's* Microcosmographia *(London, 1615). Reproduced by
permission of the Harvey Cushing/John Hay Whitney Medical Library of Yale University.*

It is immediately clear from Crooke's address to the "Worshipfull . . . Chyrurgeons" of England that he is writing in the midst of what is now called the medical marketplace, a competitive commercial field in which practitioners, both licensed and unlicensed, lettered and illiterate, vied for clients and authority.[9] The practical uses of anatomy had typically been recognized in England more by surgeons than by the theoretically grounded physicians, and earlier writers of English anatomical texts, such as Vicary and Banister, had themselves been surgeons. Crooke, too, addressed himself to an audience of surgeons, and in doing so he signaled his participation in an ongoing effort to establish a field of *learned* surgery, one that could clearly be distinguished from the work of unlettered empirics and quacks.[10] But unlike Vicary and Banister, Crooke was a physician, not a surgeon; thus, while he endeavors to make anatomical knowledge available to his unlatined audience, he is careful to indicate that their education should not lead to professional presumption. His preface seeks to balance a seemingly goodwilled (if somewhat condescending) desire to inform with an authoritative warning not to presume. Crooke explains in his address to his intended audience, "The Worshipfull Company of Barber-Chyrurgeons," that his "description of the bodie of man" was intended to "ground and establish you in the Principles and Theory and Contemplative part of your profession" (*M*, 1 r). But as much as the stated intent was to educate surgeons and thus elevate both their status and the status of their craft, it is also apparent that this was to be done only within certain limits that were, in theory at least, clearly defined. There was a hierarchy to be maintained between those who performed "manuary labour," that is, surgeons, and physicians, who "fit [their] minde[s] for greater difficulties" (*M*, 1 v).[11] Thus, though, as Banister had pointed out, the surgeon needed to know anatomy because it was impossible to treat the body effectively if you did not know anything about the parts themselves,[12] the surgeon, Crooke warned, should nonetheless "content himselfe with the limits of his profession and not usurpe upon the profession of the physitian" (ibid.).

These signs of professional competition between surgeons and physicians were part of a long-standing and larger controversy about the usefulness of making medical knowledge, whether anatomical, physiological, or pharmacological, available in the vernacular. As medical texts began to appear in English in the sixteenth century, learned physicians, educated at university and trained to understand medicine as an aspect of natural philosophy, worried that medicine would be corrupted and dangerous in the hands of the unlatined. As one physician wrote in 1566, "[E]nglishe bookes teacheth nothinge of the trewe foundation of Phisike . . . howe can it be well understanded without logike and naturall philosophie" (topics traditionally taught in Latin at university).[13] Learned medicine, of course, had always been both theoretical and practical, comprising both an intellectual system of explanation and a series of therapeutic techniques. The university curricula that prevailed from the thirteenth century emphasized the dependence of practical medical skill on established traditions of book learning; in England, it was not until the end of the seventeenth century that the medical curriculum changed from being author-based to being disease-based.[14] Writers in the vernacular, however, would have none of these claims of learning's preserves; they countered such claims with accusations of monopolistic desire, particularly against the London College of Physicians, which, founded in 1518, had had exclusive jurisdiction over physicians practicing within seven miles of London from 1523 on.[15] Though a few English texts demur, particularly on whether to translate into English the "secrets" of the female generative parts, most prefaces to English-language medical texts defend their translations as a ready way to disseminate medical knowledge, both to professional medical practitioners and (well-to-do) lay people.[16]

Thomas Elyot's *The Castel of Health* (1541 [1536]) is one of the first popular medical manuals in English and also one of the most ardent in its defense of the vernacular:

> [I]f phistions be angry, that I have wryten phisike in englyshe, let thym remember, that the grekes wrote in greke, the Romanes in latyne, Avicena . . . in Arabike, whiche were their own proper and maternal tonges. And if they had bene as moche attacked with envy and covaytise, as some now seeme to be, they wolde have devised somme particular language, with a strange syphre or fourme off letters, wherin they wold have written their science, which no man shoulde have knowen that had not professed and practised phisycke.[17]

Over 100 years later, the prolific medical popularizer Nicholas Culpeper was still arguing much the same point. In the preface to his 1649 translation of the *Pharmacopoeia Londinenisis*—the standard guide for apothecaries originally published by the Royal College of Physicians in 1618—Culpeper asserted against his detractors his ability to understand and his duty to disseminate medical recipes. Just as, he says, it is not the Cowl that makes the Munk, the shaking of the Urinal, the stroaking of the beard, Hard words, the Plush Cloak, a large House with a Monster in the first room to amaze the Patient, but deep grounded Reason, and tried Experience, that commences a Physician.[18]

Crooke's exertions were somewhat less activist than Culpeper's but like Culpeper decades later, Crooke published his work against the authority of the Bishop of London, who took particular offence at the illustrations to Book Four on the generative parts and against the explicit wishes of the College of Physicians, whose president warned that were the book to be printed without deleting the offending sections, he would himself burn whatever copies he found.[19] Crooke defied them all, had the unexpurgated book printed anyway, and defended his decision on the grounds that writing only in Latin would have undermined his high-minded purpose "to better them who do not so wel understand that language" (*M*, ii v). His goal was well achieved, since the enormous and certainly expensive text was reissued in 1616 and 1618, and went through both a second and a third edition in 1631 and 1651.

These prefatory justifications are commercial at their heart, revealing the fundamentally financial aims of both medical practitioners and booksellers, and they place the books firmly in their contemporary setting.[20] But a more extended, perhaps a more conceptual and certainly a much more ancient justification of the value of anatomy comes in Book One, a justification that Crooke borrowed from Caspar Bauhin, who, along with André du Laurens, constitutes the primary sources for Crooke's text.[21] Here the argument is less about the practice of medicine and more about its philosophical grounding. The question Crooke addresses is simply this: why is it necessary to study anatomy? Or, perhaps more precisely, why is it important to read a 1,000–page book about anatomy? Practically, of course, a surgeon who knows basic anatomy has less of a chance of butchering his patient than one who does not, but the argument is fundamentally more abstract than that and it indicates the extent to which Crooke's text is still embedded in a premodern worldview. Crooke pronounces anatomy to be the most worthy and most esteemed of all the "manie Arts full of secret and abstruse notions, deepe mysteries, and high comtemplations" (*M*, 1), because, he says, drawing on a tradition that goes back at least to Plato, in the "frame of man" there is signified "an Epitome or compend of the whole creation." "There is nothing," Crooke says, either in heaven or on earth, or in the administration of them both, not only on mans part, but which is more, on Gods also, that is not equaled, yea the divine history giveth us warrant to say, exceeded in the frame of man. (*M*, 2)

Crooke's demonstration of this commonplace that man is a microcosm resorts to equally commonplace formulas—being made in the image of God, man has the image of divine nature "most lively imprinted in his soul and in his body" (*M*, 2), and since that nature is the foundation of the whole creation, "all things are found in the body of man, which this universall world doth embrace and comprehend" (*M*, 7). Thus man encapsulates in his body the three realms of existence, the angelic, the celestial, and the sublunary:

> The Images and resemblances of which three partes, who seeth not plainly expressed, and as it were portrayed out with a curious pensill in the body of man? The head, the Castle and tower of the soule . . . is most like to the Angels or intelligencies. . . . The middle and celestiall part, is in the breast or middle venter. . . . For as in that celestiall part, the Sun is predominant, by whose motion, beames, and light, all things have their brightnesse . . . , so in the middest of the chest, the heart resideth, whose like-nesse and proportion with the Sun, is such and so great, as the ancient writers have been bolde to call the Sun, the Heart of the world, and the heart the Sunne of mans bodie. . . . Now further, who seeth not the sublunary part of the world expressed in the inferior venter or lower belly? For in it are contained the parts that are ordained for nourishment and procreation. (*M*, 6–7)

These correspondences between the micro- and macrocosm are, of course, traditional truisms, and they found the ancient idea of the great chain of being. But Crooke's understanding of man as a microcosm extends beyond these somewhat large-scale correlations. For Crooke, anatomy represents the minute particularities of the universe, its hierarchies and manifold interrelations, all of which are signified within the intricacies of man's insides. Thus, to take just a few of the many examples offered, the four humors of the body correspond to the four elements of the physical universe, with the spirit or "quintessence" "answering to the element of the starres" (*M*, 7); the "wandering planets," too, are present, with the Moon "resembled by the streaming marrow and pith of the back and braine," and Venus "proportioned in the generative parts," and "To Mercurie so variable, and withal so ingenuous, the instruments of eloquence and sweet delivery are

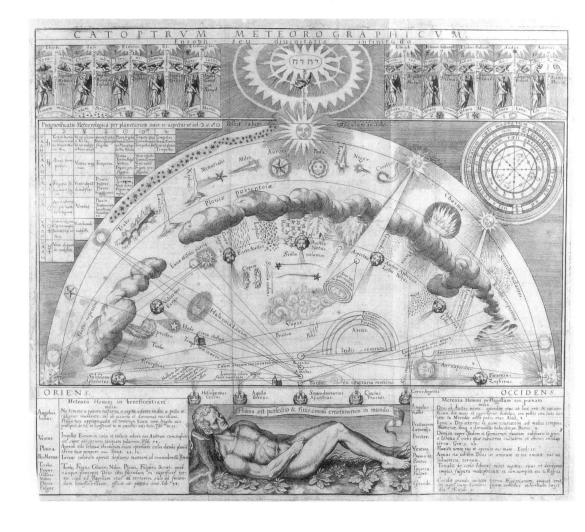

*Plate 3. From Robert Fludd,* Philosophia sacra et vere Christiana seu meterologia cosmica *(Frankfurt, 1626), the plate depicts the meteorological phenomena, both good and ill, that pervade the macrocosm; man is, as the banner proclaims, "the perfection and end of all creatures in the universe." Meteorology in the macrocosm manifests in the microsm of the human body as passions and disease. Reproduced by permission of the Harvey Cushing/John Hay Whitney Medical Library of Yale University.*

answereable" (ibid.). Not only the elements and planets but the weather, too, is limned in man's body, constituting a veritable "meterology of this little world" called man. Lightning is "shewed in the ruddie suffusions of our eyes"; thunder is replicated in "the rumbling of the guts, their croaking murmurs"; the "gathering rage of blustering windes" are "foreshewed by exhaled crudities." And the list goes on—phlegm dripping in the throat is like rain; phlegm coughed up into the throat is like hailstones; tears are like dew; shaking is like earthquakes; and kidney stones "do carry a resemblance of Mines and Mineralles" (*M*, 7–8).

These correspondences, too, are commonplace (see plate 3), although here more minutely (if not maniacally) drawn than usual. But in the context of *Microcosmographia*'s apologia for anatomy, they give weight and substance to the premise of Crooke's argument, which is essentially an interpretation of the ancient oracle of Apollo, who famously advised, "Know Thyself." Crooke concurs, but the means he proposes are less traditional than the aim; one learns to know oneself not through abstract introspection but rather by knowing one's anatomy. "This same knowledge of a mans selfe, as it is a very glorious thing, so it is also very hard and difficult. And yet by the dissection of the body, and by Anatomy, wee shall easily attaine unto this knowledge" (*M*, 11).[22] And when one knows one's self, which means one's anatomy, then one knows both the cosmos (which it epitomizes) and its Creator.

But there is a question that the neatness and familiarity of this extended argument leaves unanswered, namely, what self is implicated by anatomy? The body, Crooke says, epitomizes the created cosmos, and the body tells the self: anatomy is a species of autopsy, of self-seeing, literally. But does that suggest that the self known by the body is consonant with the cosmos? Crooke writes earlier on in Book One that the soul is a "lively resemblance of the ineffable Trinity" (*M*, 4), but he quickly shies away from the topic of the soul, knowing that he cannot "open that shrine which Nature her selfe hath veiled and sealed up from our senses" (ibid.). And anyway, the soul is not the same as the self; he does not use the words interchangeably. So what is it that gets known about the *self* when one studies anatomy? Crooke is never explicit about this, about how the self relates to the body he anatomizes in such careful detail. For Galen, I have suggested, the body tells a distributed, embodied, embedded self, a self that is literally, materially consonant with the cosmos. But for Crooke. . . ?

As a product of Christian culture, Crooke could not espouse all aspects of Galen's somatic system. He could not, for example, comfortably leave unanswered the question of the psyche's materiality; for him, the psyche, which he understood to be the soul, is "incorporeall, immortall, [and] immutable" (ibid.). This was a truth "unknowne to the ancient Philosophers, who groaped but in the darke" (ibid.).[23] Crooke's Christianized version of the Galenic psyche is typical of the syncretic nature of his text, which assays to modulate pagan with Christian, ancient with modern. But this effort at reconciliation presented him as well as other revivers of ancient learning with the problem of maintaining Galen's authority in matters anatomical and physiological while acknowledging the evidence of the modern anatomy theater. That Galen needed "correction" or emendation on questions related to religion and philosophy had long been recognized and was readily explained by his paganism; Maimonides had already established in the twelfth century that Galen's "opinions ought to be followed only in medicine and in nothing else."[24] The challenging issue was not how to handle his explicit statements of philosophy; it was how to preserve the hegemony of the Galenic *body* when Vesalius and others, though still writing within a Galenic paradigm, were nonetheless pointing to his explicit anatomical "mistakes." It is this conceptual challenge that provides the context for understanding Crooke's permutations of the Galenic person because it is only by recognizing how ardently he attempts to adhere to the Galenic body, even in the face of growing objections to it, that we can see how deeply he diverges from Galen in matters of the self.

In the most comprehensive anatomy printed in English before Crooke's, John Banister solves the problem of reconciliation in a fairly radical way, by arguing that bodies have to be understood locally both in time and place, and that challenges to Hippocratic and Galenic anatomy therefore do not truly threaten the authority of the ancients. Though he admits that the words of Galen and Hippocrates "are not as Gospell in all things" (*HM*, 101 r), Banister argues that Galen and Hippocrates fully deserve the "excellencie we ascribe" to them, that none "hath bene their equals," and that "from their fountains flow the springing streames, that nourishe Phisicke for ever" (*HM*, Bii r). He further asserts that "what good thing soever we have, or atcheive, we are to consecrate the same unto their honor and prayse." The reason then that they are so much challenged "these days . . . especially in the partes of mans body" is that "ech age hath his tyme, eche nation his nature, and ech nature his property" (ibid.). There is, it seems, no single, universal model of the human form. To demonstrate this truth, Banister points to the obvious fact that we no longer live as long as Biblical persons did, and then he rehearses the astonishing variety of bodily forms throughout the world known from histories both ancient and modern—for example, the Macrocephali of Asia, who have elongated heads, or "them who with one leg cover their whole body," which he claims is a "familiar syght" in India (*HM*, Biii r). The point is that "sundry mutations do happen" in the body of man, which he knows as well from his own experience in dissection; he has twice seen a liver divided into lobes, an anatomical arrangement that is consonant with ancient authority but is rejected by modern anatomists (*HM*, Biiii v). The differences among bodies he therefore imputes not to the mistakes of the ancients but to the "varieties of regions and change of times" (ibid.). For Banister, at least in his explicit defense of Galen, the body is a mutable, adaptable construct, and the knowledge he offers to the "fellowly Fraternitie of Chirurgians in London" must therefore be understood as localized only.

Crooke takes a tellingly different tack in his defense of Galen, which allows him to acknowledge modern controversies while not at all relativizing the knowledge he gets from his ancient authority. He does admit that it is wrong to believe that the art of medicine is "already perfected and consummated by those which went before us" and he argues that it is not acceptable to "limit [one's] noble wits within other mens bounds." Still, he says, the foundation and framework of the "building" of bodily knowledge was set by the ancients, so that "now if any ornaments be added, they must be fitted thereunto: wherefore we have labored to bring all the subtleties and novell inventions of the later writers, to the Touch-stone of the ancients Monuments" (*M*, 36–37). For Crooke, the framework of the ancients, by whom he means primarily Hippocrates and Galen, is paramount. Their body is the only and real one, so that any changes now deemed necessary must be "fitted" to the already existent and solid structure. Changes are "ornamental," rather than foundational.

We can see Crooke applying his rather conservative mode of syncretism in his treatment of the *rete mirabile*, the "marvelous network" of arteries that Galen had asserted exists in man—wrongly as it turned out. The rete mirabile is a complex arrangement of arteries at the base of the skull said by Galen to be the structure that allowed the production of psychic pneuma (translated as the animal spirit in English Galenism). Blood, traveling through the rete mirabile, would have to slow down as it negotiated the complexities of the network; in the time of its sojourn there, the blood would be further refined into a more airy substance that, in its final elaboration in the ventricles of the brain, would become psychic pneuma. This substance, as we saw in the last chapter, traveled from the brain through the nerves to the body parts and thereby made possible both sensation and voluntary motion—cognitive activities that, according to Galen, take place in the parts themselves. Psychic pneuma was, in Galen, the means by which  perception was distributed to the parts, so that the subjectification of the parts was not mere rhetoric but rather indicated the ability of the parts to recognize their wants.

In 1522, Giacomo Berengario de Carpi determined that the rete mirabile does not exist in humans, and Vesalius, at least by the time he published the *Fabrica* in 1543, concurred.[25] But in an intellectual move typical of the time, instead of doubting the bit of Galenic physiology that had depended on what was for them a disproved bit of Galenic anatomy, both Berengario and Vesalius preserved the idea of psychic pneuma but relegated its production to other parts. Galen, they determined, had dissected apes and other animals more than he had men; his anatomical errors could therefore be attributed to his willingness to generalize across kinds. But this methodological error did not jeopardize his overall theory— psychic pneuma was still elaborated from the blood, only now the process took place entirely in the brain; the rete mirabile was not needed to elaborate the blood before it reached the brain. Crooke's response was even more reactionary; he simply denied the denial. Against Vesalius, Bauhin claimed that he had himself seen the rete mirabile in many of his human dissections, and Crooke simply accepted his testimony. Galen's rete mirabile *did* exist in humans.

Given how strenuously Crooke tries to preserve Galen's authority, it is all the more relevant that the self implicated in the body he discursively anatomizes differs so deeply from his ancient source. Renaissance scholars attending both to Crooke's elaborate explication of microcosmic man as well to his faithful presentation of Galenic bio-medicine tend to view *Microcosmographia*, rightly I think, as the apogee of Renaissance medicine—a text composed and compiled at the apex of the Galenic revival and aware of, but not yet wholly affected by, the numerous challenges to Galenism that, by the end of the seventeenth century, would see the tradition wane and finally die out. But the text works changes on its Galenic inheritance, and not just in its inconsistent acceptance of the work of the moderns. The sense of self is different; the Galenic body still tells the self, but no longer a Galenic self. As a close reading of Crooke's prose will show, in place of the distributed, embodied Galenic self, we get a self that is separate from and presides over the body; we get, in short, the supervenient, disembodied self of the early modern world, one that, as we shall see, is decidedly, if implicitly, gendered exclusively as male.

■  Crooke's permutations of traditional Galenism can readily be seen in his treatment of the anatomy of the stomach and the physiology of digestion. Both are thoroughly Galenic, deriving, via du Laurens, from Galen's *On the Usefulness of the Parts of the Body.* Like Galen, Crooke describes a teleological body; but if the overarching premise of Galen's ancient teleology is that the parts are made by the prescience of Nature so as best to fulfill their own particular functions and thereby promote the overall well-being of the organism, the telos Crooke's body serves is more emphatically that of a separable and ever-present self whose ends are served by, but are not coextensive with, the ends of the body.

Discussing the placement of the stomach in the abdomen, Crooke talks as if about a loving relationship, a considerate interaction among internal parts:

> It lyeth for the most part of it in the left Hypochondrium . . . because here it had most roome, and againe for the more commodious implantation of the upper mouth, by which it receiveth the meate; moreover, to give way unto the Liver which takes up the right side; and lastly, with the Spleene to helpe to balance the body against the Liver. . . . On the right side, the upper and forepart of it lyeth under the hollownesse of the Liver, and by it is embraced, whereby his heate is cherished. . . . Behind it are, the backbone as a strong and thicke defence, and the Muscles of the Loynes as a soft bed with fat growing thereto for his better repose, which also doe adde warmth unto it. (*M*, 117)

The central organ of the abdomen, the stomach finds its place among other parts that defend, warm, and embrace it. The other parts seem here to be built to serve the needs of the stomach and to provide for its comfort. The somatic economy of the abdomen seems localized, nearly self-sufficient. But Crooke quickly makes it clear that the stomach is not the central show, that it, in turn, is built to serve a greater whole:

> On the outside it is smooth, plaine and white: within when it is knit or gathered together, it is rugous or rugged (as we see in Tripes) and reddish. It is hollow, and his hollownesse of all other parts the most ample, that it might receive sufficient quantity of meate and drinke, least for our nourishment we should be constrained to bee always eating; now, when it is once full or satisfied, wee may have leisure for other businesse, whilst all the meate taken at a meale, be digested and distributed. (*M*, 118)

The general scheme is thoroughly Galenic, the part functioning precisely as an *organ*, an instrument acting on behalf of the whole. But Crooke's rhetoric tweaks the implied telos: whereas in Galen, the parts work as if autonomously but for the sake of an inseparable psychosomatic unity, here the part serves an abstracted whole, something conceptually separable from the body. The shape and structure of the stomach are such that "we" are able to get on with business other than eating, *we* should not be "constrained" by the body; luckily, the body is made to give us liberty to act on our "leisure for other businesse." The flesh seems providentially made to serve the self, and this assumption of subservience gets registered through the attribution of agency. Crooke gives the active verbs to "us": *we* eat, *we* need leisure for business; the stomach itself is passive. This passivity even resonates in the restricted meaning of *satisfied*: whereas the Latinate word can indicate what we would call conscious contentment, its anglicized cognate, *full*, signifies merely a material measure.

What I am pointing to here is a tendency to posit a subject of a particular kind through subtle rhetorical formulations. That subject is figured as being both superior and prior to the part described—it is supervenient. In this passage, that subject, the collective *we* of humanity, is an entity that deserves to be unconstrained by the body, that needs its leisure, that has business to conduct, and that, happily, is served by a body described in terms of inert matter.

This not an incidental occurrence in Crooke's text. In the act of digestion, agency is routinely given to a posited person rather than to the part, as it would be in traditional Galenic physiology. Thus, for example, when Crooke explains that a thick mesh of "membranous and nervous" fibers helps the stomach's ability to expand and contract, he warns that "in whomsoever the body of the stomach is thin, such men do worse concoct their meat, than they that have it fleshy and thicke" (*M*, 119). Men, not stomachs, concoct their meat. Similarly, when Crooke explains why the *cardia*, the sensitive opening of the stomach from the esophagus, is so thick, he presents a body part that is passive in relation to a supervenient person:

> Thicker also it is than the other [opening in the stomach leading to the small intestines], least it should be violated when it is constrained to receiye hard, thicke, and unchewed gobbets, such as hunger-bitten folke do with great ravenousnesse swallow downe and devoure. (*M*, 118)

Here, the part is at the mercy of the bad behavior of "hunger-bitten folk," who foolishly choose to swallow "unchewed gobbets" of food. The stomach itself is "constrained" to suffer their choices.

In Galen, by contrast, the parts are always active, endowed with "godlike faculties" that promote their "well-tempered actions" (*UP*, 205). Galen's introductory description of "the parts of nutrition" conveys well this sense of their active agency. The stomach, he writes, is a

> storehouse, a work of divine, not human art, [which] receives all the nutriment and subjects the food to its first elaboration, without which it would be useless and of no benefit whatever to the animal. For just as workmen skilled in preparing wheat cleanse it of any earth, stones, or foreign seeds mixed with it that would be harmful to the body, so the faculty of the stomach thrusts downward anything of that sort, but makes all the rest of the material, that is naturally good, still better and distributes it to the veins extending to the stomach and intestines.
>
> Just as city porters carry the wheat cleaned in the storehouse to some public bakery of the city where it will be baked and made fit for nourishment, so these veins carry the nutriment already elaborated in the stomach up to a place for concoction common to the whole animal, a place which we call the liver. (*UP*, 204)

Whereas for Crooke men concoct their food into chyle, the parts rhetorically placed to serve the supervenient person, for Galen, stomachs themselves do the concocting, "subject[ing] food to its first elaboration." The rhetorical focus in Galen is on the intentional activity of the parts, which are likened to skilled workmen and industrious porters, interactive agents in a whole that exists conceptually as an effect of their efforts. The animal, in other words, is compared to a well-run city, as an entity that cannot be understood as either prior to or separable from its constitutive components, which are the agential parts.

Crooke's rhetorical formulations preserve Galen's basic anatomy but they reconfigure the sense of the person whose anatomy is being described. It is important, then, that when Crooke does grant typical Galenic subjectivity to a part—as, for example, in the stomach's ability to perceive its want—he is careful to posit a person over and above it. Describing the upper orifice of the stomach, Crooke writes:

> This Orifice because of the aboundance of sinnewes [nerves] that it receyveth, is of most exquisite sense, that it might feele its owne want; which sence of want stirreth up the appetite, that the creature might address himselfe to provide for more meat and drinke to satisfie it. (*M*, 118)

This seems quite similar to Galen's discussion of the same material in *On the Usefulness of the Parts*. The stomach is endowed with the capacity to feel its own want; at some level, the stomach itself is granted an *awareness* of its need. But there is a difference, too: in Galen, the appetite occurs in the stomach itself; in Crooke, the stomach feels its want but the locus of the appetite is left unspecified, and it is the creature as a whole that acts with intention, that addresses itself to provide meat and drink. Whatever mode of awareness is granted to the stomach, the prose grants a higher level of agency to the whole creature.

When the pattern recurs a few pages later, Crooke erases any ambiguity about the site of cognitive perception and affect. Still describing the *cardia*, Crooke focuses on the function of its abundance of sinews, or nerves:

> [I]t seemeth to be made altogether of sinews; from the aboundance of which, it hath most exquisite sence to stirre up and awake the sence of the want of nourishment, which sence ariseth from suction; there is the seat of the appetite; and to this onely part [the stomach] hath nature given the sence of want or of animal hungry. (*M*, 121)

Of all the organs, the stomach alone has the capacity to sense its want, but "we" are what feels hungry; the stomach's admitted "sence of want" gets altogether absorbed in and transferred to the "we" who feel both the inner contraction and the sense of hunger. And that "we" takes over the rest of the paragraph:

> For if we should not feele a kinde of molestation upon the utter and absolute exsuction of our nourishment till there be a supply made, we should by degrees be extinguished being affamished before we were aware. (*M*, 121–22)

We—something other than the body—feel the body as an object of our affective perception. This is not Galen's distributed cognition but rather the emergence of a top-down manager, of subjectivity acting independently and purposefully on information supplied by subservient parts. The teleology still exists but now we have a body teleologically constructed to serve "us" and "our" needs.

Crooke, in fact, is most explicit about the hierarchy between matter and self when he is most explicit about what seems dangerously close to being the selfhood of matter. Discussing "Whether the Upper Part of the Stomach be the Seate of the Appetite," Crooke explains that there are three kinds of nourishment necessary for the preservation of life: air, meat, and drink. He then continues:

> But because there can be no nourishment without Appetite, Nature hath dispensed to every part a certaine desire, whereby as by goades they are pricked forward to draw and sucke into themselves convenient and familiar aliment. But this desire in the particular parts is without sense, for they feele not neither perceive when they draw or sucke such convenient aliment. Wherefore, lest the parts should pine away when they are exhausted and as it were hunger-starved, nature hath framed one part of exquisite and perfect sence, which alone fore-apprehending the suction and so the want of the rest, should stirre up the creatures to provide and cooke their nourishment for them. For if the sense of this suction or traction were in every part, then in the time of affamishment or thirst they would perpetually languish, and so the creature leade his life in perpetual disease. (*M*, 169)

So the stomach, like other parts, has the desire for nourishment but, unlike other parts, the stomach also has the ability to perceive its desire, which makes it able to apprehend in advance the needs of the other parts. The stomach here seems to have a faculty that we might more comfortably (if anachronistically) ascribe to *consciousness*—the ability to "fore-apprehend" a need and modify present actions based on predictions about the future. But even so, this capacity is clearly subjugated to the creature's need to "leade his life." Crooke makes the hierarchy explicit at the end of the section:

> [W]ee must not here forget that though this appetite of the stomacke bee with sence, yet it is not ioyned with knowledge or discretion. (*M*, 170)

Body parts may have certain attributes of subjectivity, but Crooke wants it to be unambiguously understood that they do not possess those that characterize a human subject.

Crooke's pattern of superimposing a subject on the seeming subjectivity of matter is not restricted to his discussions of the stomach and its processes. It is even more apparent in his treatment of the penis, commonly called the "yard." Again, the starkest example emerges at the moment of greatest personification of the part. Crooke is describing the structure of the penis, specifically the "canals" within it through which the spirits flow to cause an erection:

> These bodies are also rare and porous, that they might suddenly bee filled with spirites and with venall and arteriall bloud when the yeoman is irritated or incensed; and his violence being appeased, the same spirits and blood being partly dissipated and partly returned into the vessels, settle and shorted again. For if the member were always strong and stiffe, it would be a great hinderance to men in many labours of this life, especially such as are violent, and beside it selfe would bee always subject to mischiefes, even as the arme or hand would be if it were continually streatched forth. (*M*, 211–12)

Here, the "yeoman" penis seems to be emphatically subjectified; it is not only personified by name but gets described according to its moods (irritated, incensed, and appeased). The penis seems to be a hardworking laborer though a potentially dangerous one, given its propensity to anger and violence. Yet, lest the danger be a true threat rather than merely a rhetorical one, the prose puts the yeoman in its place, beneath the subject it serves—the penis settles down, shortens, and lets men get on with the "many labours of this life." Of course, a yeoman is a man, but a man defined by and thus in some sense synonymous with his labor. "Men," by contrast, are not conceptually contained by labor. Labor is something men perform; it is not definitional of who they are.

In noting the rhetorical imposition of the supervening self as a counter to a subjectified part, I find myself again in disagreement with the editors of the rightly admired and influential collection of essays *The Body in Parts* who argue that the "individuated agencies" of body parts are unique and telling features of the early modern period and that the period's attention to the meaning of the parts "attest[s] to the emergence in early modern culture of what may be called a new aesthetic of the part, which is to say an aesthetic that did not demand or rely upon the reintegration of the part into a predetermined whole."[26] By contrast, I am arguing that what is *traditional* about these medical texts is precisely their attention to and granting of what we would consider agency to body parts, that this was entirely normative, and that what is *new* in Crooke is the insistence on an a priori and supervening self. Crooke's basic anatomy and physiology are Galenic, but his rhetorical tropings add what is neither present in Galen nor, more importantly, *necessary* in his system. The early modern subject—self-aware, goal-directed, and free from the burdens of the body—emerges in Crooke's text as an assumption of its rhetorical formulations, a being putatively grounded in sinew and bone but built in fact from the capacities of prose.

■ If writing about the body always implicates assumptions about the self, it would make sense to consider how Crooke fashions bodies that are marked particularly as female, for the body I have been considering so far, though figured as ungendered, is really the male body taken as the norm. That the normative body was implicitly male in ancient Galenism is evinced perhaps most obviously by the homology Galen proposed between the male and female reproductive parts. As Crooke explained, the female had roughly the same anatomy as the male but, because of her lesser heat, the parts existed inside her body where they could retain warmth rather than outside, as they did on the warmer and more perfect males. Women have

> all those parts belonging to generation which men have, although in these they appear outward . . . in those they are for want of heate retained within. (*M*, 216)

This one-sex model of the body, in which the female essentially has no existence independent of the male but is, rather, its involuted form, was not uniformly accepted in the early modern period, and Crooke includes in his discussion of reproductive anatomy some of the contemporary debates about its adequacy as a descriptive model of the sexes.[27] Yet he does not question the assumption of the normativity of the male body or the sense that the female body has a conceptually separate existence only insofar as it has specific reproductive capacities. What Crooke presents as the universal body is really gendered as male, from which the female exists as an inferior deviation.

A similar pattern pertains in Crooke's inscription of selves: though what I am calling the supervenient self is not explicitly gendered, it is in fact a specifically masculine model. This is demonstrated by Crooke's rather different treatment of the specifically female body; when discussing female parts, Crooke does not provide the supervenient self, as he does with the normative (male) parts. The female generative parts are insistently personified, but with no stable self to contain them. The asymmetry is evident when we compare how Crooke differently attributes modes of freedom to the normative male and specifically female bodies. Recall the good-natured efforts of the stomach, which, by concocting food for the whole somatic system, allow us to be "at leisure" to perform our (presumably non-somatic) business. In discussing female anatomy, by contrast, Crooke assigns a rather different version of liberty—the womb, he explains, is not immobile; rather, it is loose, free and at liberty, that it might better be distended in women with child, and in coition when the desire of conception is [it] might more freely move, now upward then downeward and open it selfe to the end of the yard. (*M*, 223)

Aware that the womb is "held stedfast by membranous ligaments that connect it to the muscles of the loines" (ibid.), Crooke, along with almost everyone else at the time, was adamant in denying the ancient (though also anciently discredited) idea that the womb was an animal, moving at will in a woman's body and causing all manner of distress.[28] But though he is confident that the womb is "not like a gadding creature that moveth out of one place into another" (*M*, 224), he seems easily ready to assign to the organ aspects of agency—being free and at liberty—that he elsewhere assigns to some supervenient "us." And yet the womb, unlike *us*, holds only a middling mode of liberty; it is free to open itself to the yard but not free enough to move wherever it wants. The womb possesses, then, a rather particular type of liberty. It is free to be self-ruled but only as long as that rule directs it to serve its procreative function. The womb seems in fact to epitomize the paradoxical position of the female in early modern patriarchy: she is not slavish, not without mind (not, in other words, an animal) but expected by the patent validity of patriarchy to consent willingly to her role within it. William Whately neatly exemplifies the paradox in his 1617 advice book for young women; in order for a marriage to thrive, a woman must, *of her own volition*, acknowledge her inferiority:

Whosoever therefore doth desire or purpose to be a good wife, or to live comfortably, let her set down this conclusion within her soul: mine husband is my superior, my better; he hath authority and rule over me.[29]

A woman's free will is asserted, but only insofar as it directs her to be subservient to her husband.[30]

This tendency to articulate the womb in terms of a social norm for the female is everywhere apparent in Crooke. The pattern partakes of the Galenic tendency to animate the parts, to grant them modes of what to us seem aspects of higher-order agency and affect, but rather than constructing alongside the animated part a conscientious and mindful self that presides over and above it (as we see in descriptions of the normative, male body), the text personifies the womb as an unruly part that overtakes the possibility of a superimposed, freely determining self.

The most obvious instance of this pattern appears in the multiplicity of names used to refer to the organ itself.[31] Though he most commonly uses the word *womb*, Crooke explains that Aristotle called the organ the "Field of Nature" because it is the place of producing "new off-spring." Hippocrates called it "gyne" and Pliny called it "locus," because it is "the place of a woman"; but it is also, he says, called "mater" or "the mother, because it is the mother of the infant" (*M*, 222). The names "field of nature" and "locus" or "gyne" refer to the womb's physiological and anatomical function; to call it "the mother," however, is not only explicitly to personify it but also to attribute to it a role more reasonably reserved for a woman. Personifying the womb as the mother, in other words, allows an easy slippage between part and person; if the womb-as-mother is the mother of the infant, then what role does what *we* call the mother have in conception, pregnancy, and birth? By contrast, no such slippage pertains to male anatomy; the penis in its labors might be described as a yeoman, but it is never referred to as a "man," let alone as a "father."

The logic of this slippage consistently directs Crooke's engagement of the womb's anatomical position and physiological function. Like the stomach, the womb is closely surrounded by other parts in the body's interior and, like the stomach, it lies on one of its neighbors as on "a pillow" (*M*, 223). But if the stomach partakes of a social economy in which it provides nourishment and receives tender attention in turn, the womb, at least in relation to its surroundings, needs rather more protection. It is, Crooke explains, "compassed about as with strong rampires for defence, with the share bones before, the great bone behinde, and the hanch bones on either side" (ibid,). Thus protected by the rigid structure of the surrounding bones, the womb gets further protection from the soft parts nearest it, the bladder and the right gut, so that it might not be "hurt" by the hardness of the bones behind it and might have a"bulwarke to defend it" in the front. In this context, the womb seems less an effective member of the bodily order than a helpless creature in need of defense.

Somewhat paradoxically, this slippage of woman and womb is most apparent anatomically in precisely those descriptions provided to disprove the idea that the womb can wander about the body causing havoc, like an animal. Crooke explains that the ligaments that hold the womb to the loins are "like to Bridles" that "do hold in the womb" (ibid.); the womb, he says, is not an animal, but rather "rideth as a moored Ship in a Tempest betweene her Anchors" (ibid.). Though explicitly denying the animality of the womb, Crooke's similes nevertheless attest to the womb's dangerous tendency to roam. For surely, though a ship could never be mistaken for an animal, it certainly would sail away in a tempest were it not securely moored, and one uses bridles precisely to keep animals under control. Like the stomach, the womb is endowed with attractive, retentive, and expulsive faculties (in this sense, the two differ only in terms of *what* they attract, retain, and expel) but, unlike the stomach, the womb must be fastened to its proper place by four strong ligaments. It has to be bridled because its nature leads it to err. In a period when conduct books advised husbands to rein in their wandering wives, the bridled womb seems an easy conflation.

Crooke routinely makes this same move, telescoping manifold constructions of the female (defenseless, erring, desirous, yet industrious if properly controlled) into depictions of the womb. This is especially apparent in his description of the womb's role in conception. In standard Galenic fashion, the womb by nature desires and longs after seed (so much so, in fact, that one common cause of female illness was understood to be the womb's lack of the refreshment that the seed provides) (*M*, 296). Once the seed of both parents arrives at the mouth of the womb, the womb draws the seed to its bottom through the aegis of its attractive faculty and then it mingles the seed together; after that, Crooke tells us,

> the womb, which is the most noble and almost divine Nurse, gathereth and contracteth it self [until] . . . there is no empty or void place left therein. And this it doth as being greedy to conteyne and to cherish, we say to Conceive the seed. Moreoever, least the geniture thus layd up should issue forth again; the mouth or orifice of the wombe is so exquisitely shut and locked up that it will not admit the point of a needle. The wombe rowzeth and raiseth upp the sleepy and lurking power of the seeds, and that which was before but potential, it bringeth into act. This action of the wombe we properly call Conception. (*M*, 262–63)

When all is working right, the womb as divine nurse is "greedy" for the work it is supposed to perform; the "mother," acting as a good mother, cherishes the seed it draws to it and rouses its sleepy potential into action. In the properly functioning world of home economics, then, the womb is a hardworking housewife:

> The Generative faculty which before lay steeped, drowsie, and as it were intercepted in the seede, being now raised up by the heat and inbred propriety of the wombe breaketh out into act, as raked Cinders into a luculent flame. (*M*, 263)

Rousing the sleepy, acting with propriety, even raking the cinders by a cauldron where a conception is cooking, the womb performs its work with dutiful efficiency.

If in conceiving and nourishing the child, the womb models the perfect housewife and mother, at the time of birth, it (she) acts in its (her) own best interest. The causes of parturition were not clearly agreed upon in the early seventeenth century, with some writers attributing the cause primarily to the womb's strong muscular contractions and others pointing to the efforts of the infant. In Crooke, parturition is a combined effort, something like a household mini-drama, in which the violent struggles of the infant are pitted against the mother's, that is, the womb's, tolerance for abuse:

> Now when as the mother is not able to supply unto the Infant either the ayre whereby it liveth in sufficient quantity through the narrow umbilical arteries, or other nourishment by the umbilical veines, whereby it might be increased and refrigerated, the Infant then as it were undertaking of himselfe a beginning of motion, striveth to free himselfe from the prison and dungeon wherein he was restrained; kicking therefore he breaketh the membranes wherein he was inwrapped, and arming himselfe with strong violence maketh way for his inlargement with all the strength and contention that he may.
>
> This contention and distention the wombe ill brooking, and besides being overburthened with the waight of the Infant now growne, striveth to lay downe her loade, and with all her strength by that expulsive faculty wherewith she is especially furnished she rouzeth up her self, and with violence thrusteth her guest out of possession of his true inheritance. (*M*, 269)

Parturition is a joint venture of two agents working in their own self-interest, but the players are not evenly paired. One, the infant, is a person fashioned as an ideal(ized) and independent hero, "undertaking" a difficult venture, "striv[ing]" to free himself from a life-threatening "prison," arming himself with violence to emerge into the light. The other is a more passive and long-suffering body part fashioned as a woman fed up with and "overburdened" by a guest who has outstayed his welcome. She too acts with intention and violence, but the "she" who so acts remains an organ, not an agent-to-be in the world.

And what of the odd last phrase? The womb thrusts the infant out of possession of his true inheritance: the womb is figured as the infant's inheritance, the organ that "conceived" him his rightful possession, of which he is robbed. There is a murky logic here but one that seems to suggest a telling inversion that suits the emerging hierarchy between person and parts: the point of origin, though personified, is (merely) a part and thus can be understood to be rightly possessed by the full-fledged person it produces. Even when personified, even when acting in self-interest, the womb serves the coalescing conditions of possessive individualism—the male self no longer coterminus with but rightly in possession of a body.

Helkiah Crooke's *Microcosmographia* thus fulfills its promise to make anatomy the means to know the self. But the gendered selves thereby known are not symmetrically drawn. For both, the body is the ground, the material basis of their conceptual construction, but for men, the body forms the basis of and serves a supervenient self, whereas for women, a definitional body part becomes the telescoped site for a self that never clearly or consistently rises above it. Both models of the self are founded in the Galenic body, in the Galenic system of anatomy and physiology, and both make ample use of Galenic rhetoric of subjectified parts and powers. But both are also rhetorically contoured so as to write fundamental changes in the Galenic understanding of the self—the male because it substitutes supervenience for a distributed and embodied version of the self; the female because it dispenses with distribution and localizes an attenuated agency in a single organ. Neither model is determined by Galenic bio-medicine; they arise instead from the particular tropings of Crooke's rhetoric. Crooke's *Microcosmographia*, then, accomplishes more than its stated intent to describe the body of man and bring the most up-to-date Galenic learning to a wide English readership. It brings something more, something more subtle but also more lasting— an asymmetrical sense of the self that identifies the male with persons and the female with the womb.

## 3 / Fixing the Female:

### Books of Practical Physic for Women

I N 1636, THE PHYSICIAN JOHN SADLER PUBLISHED
*The Sicke Womans Private Looking-Glasse, wherein methodically are handled all uterine affects, or diseases arising from the wombe, enabling Women to informe the Physitian about the cause of their griefe.*[1] A primer on the diagnosis and treatment of
women's diseases, Sadler's text indicates by its title the essence of its intent: carrying on the familiar trope of knowing the body to know the self, Sadler invites
the sick woman to look into his medical tract as into a mirror to see herself. What
she will see there, however, as his title suggests, are not the outward signs of
her illness but rather the inward and single source of her "griefe," her womb. If
it is one's self one sees in a mirror, Sadler proposes that a sick woman's self is her
womb. Thirty years later the preface to another popular medical tract, *Mulierum
amicus: Or, the Womans Friend*, conveyed a similar idea in more elaborate terms.
Countering the efforts of proud and malicious men who have striven to keep
medical knowledge about women to themselves, Nicholas Sudell, the author of
the tract, will be "the womans friend," as his title tells us, offering assistance in
the form of medical therapies—herbal, chemical, clysters, emetics—that he will
teach his readers carefully to carry out.[2] But over and above the specific details
of his proffered medical advice, Sudell tells his audience of "noble ladies and
gentlewomen" that his purpose is "to further your knowledge . . . [of] those
things which you understand and see not (through the Pride and Malice of men)
[so that] you may apprehend and perceive 1. what you are. 2 what liable unto.
And 3. what assistance you have" (*MA*, A3 r). Practical physic ("what assistance
you have") relies on an understanding of particular vulnerabilities ("what liable
unto"), which in turn relies on an awareness of essence ("what you are"). The

practice of medicine, says Sudell, must be grounded in some conceptual frame-work that defines what a woman is, and that, he is quick to aver, inheres in "how you stand distinct from man." Perhaps not surprisingly, Sudell finds that distinction to reside in the womb, and *Mulierum amicus*, like *The Sicke Womans Private Looking-Glasse*, therefore, focuses on that one organ—its functions, its dis-eases, and, especially, what remedies are available to treat it.

Two models of woman operate in uneasy tension in both Sadler's title and Sudell's prefatory remarks. There is for each an implied reader, a woman who takes up the looking glass or picks up a book as a trusted friend, a woman of coherent intention and agency, able to act in her best interest and participate in the process of maintaining or regaining her health. But there is also in these texts her medically conceived counterpart, the thing she sees in the looking glass, the thing that her "friend" tells her she essentially is, and this is the womb. Nei-ther Sadler nor Sudell tends to the unresolved tension between the two mod-els of woman their texts endorse, between the implied agential woman, as reader or patient, and the abstracted medical conception of the body part she *really* is. In this chapter I want to consider the range of implicit tensions and embedded anxieties characterizing medical knowledge about women suggested by these texts. By looking at two of the most popular early modern guides to women's healthcare—the first, Eucharius Rösslin's *The Byrth of Mankynde*, published in two different editions, in 1540 and 1545, and the second, Nicholas Culpeper's *Directory for Midwives*, published roughly 100 years later, in 1651—along with conventional advice about Galenic treatments for women's ailments, I want to show how books written to fix women's bodies cannot themselves get a clear fix on the female self . . . unless it is conceived as a womb.[3]

■ When the first English text on women's healthcare was published in 1540, there was no learned consensus on questions relating to the particularities of women's anatomy and physiology. Medical and natural philosophical questions about women, their constitution, their role in generation, their vulnerability to particular ailments, had, of course, been widely commented on in medieval manuscript compilations, and certain large-scale areas of agreement had begun to emerge in the later Middle Ages, for example, on the male's active, formative role in conception.[4] But the consensus was evident more in terms of the ques-tions that were routinely asked than the specific answers that were offered. What was to be best understood as the defining feature of the female was a standard question in scholastic commentary, for example, but opinions varied on whether the better answer was the uterus specifically or the female's generally cooler temperament.[5] Similarly, the function of the menses was considered to be key to women's health but whether the monthly flow was best understood as a shedding of healthful but excessive blood or as a purgation of a dangerous poison that had the power to wilt grass and cloud mirrors varied among authors and commentators.[6] Frequently enough, these contradictory ideas about the female body coexisted with equally contradictory ideas about women's nature. The idea that the uterus was the central feature of the female, for example, fit neatly with the idea of woman as a passive vessel in generation. In a series of often-copied (and eventually often-reprinted) illustrations depicting the positions of the fetus in the womb, for example, the womb is presented as an inverted jar, independent of the maternal body (see plate 4 on page 77). As many have noted, these illustrations suggest not only a metonymy of womb and woman but, by way of that metonymy, the idea that the woman/womb is a passive holding place for a fetus generated by other means.[7] Yet equally common during the Middle Ages was the Galenically derived homology between the womb and the penis; women and men have the same generative organs but women, because of their lesser heat, carry theirs on the inside. Though surely in some manner lesser, the womb in this analogy takes on the more active associations of the male generative organ. And this activeness is further enforced by the Galenic idea of the womb's appetitive faculty; the womb actively craves seed, embraces it, and can cause somatic havoc if not satisfied. Though at conceptual odds, the configurations of the womb as both active and passive coexisted throughout the late Middle Ages.

Early modern tracts on women's healthcare generally and on childbearing specifically perpetuate this eclecticism. Sometimes an author will confidently claim current knowledge to have surpassed some foolishness of medieval beliefs, as when Thomas Raynalde, for example, derides as "shamefull lies and slaunders" the medieval idea that the menses are the "refuce, drosse, and vilar part" of the blood, but, as a group, early modern writers do not come any closer to consensus than do medieval writers.[8] If anything, over the course of the sixteenth and seventeenth centuries, knowledge about women's bodies gets increasingly uncertain in these popular tracts, with authors readily offering up lists of questions to which they do not know the answers or which they deem unnecessary to the pragmatic issues of practical physic.

This uncertainty attending medical knowledge about women resonates in different ways over the course of the early modern period. As we will see, in the 1545 edition of *The Byrth of Mankynde*, the uncertainty about women's somatic nature reverberates in a palpable anxiety about the prospect of making medical knowledge about women available to a wide reading public. Thomas Raynalde is adamant that he offers the work with the most honorable of intentions, but medical knowledge about women seems too troubled a topic for him to be able to control its uses. Explicit concern with audience is not as evident one hundred years later in Culpeper's popular manual, perhaps because by the mid-seventeenth century, vernacular manuals had become more widespread, and worried warnings against illicit readings had become routine. For Culpeper, the issue is more specifically connected to the medical models themselves. As Galenic learning fell increasingly under attack, its models for understanding the relations between the sexes were similarly questioned. Yet, rather paradoxically, although Culpeper reasonably questions the medical models, he is all the more certain that they express an immutable hierarchy between the sexes that denies agential personhood to the "lesser" of the two. Finally, in the selected therapeutics I will consider, the unspoken assumption subtending all the texts emerges rather explicitly—the topic cannot safely be touched, the patient cannot fully be a person, because a woman is not one *possessed* of a womb but rather one who *is* a womb, a person coextensive not with the body, but with a body part.

■ The burgeoning market for bio-medical literature in English in the sixteenth and seventeenth centuries was characterized more commonly by popular books of practical physic like Sadler's and Sudell's than by the weighty learning of Helkiah Crooke's biophilosophy. Although *Microcosmographia* was reprinted several times during the first half of the seventeenth century, commercial publication catered more avidly to books both cheaper and more specifically focused on therapeutics. By the beginning of the seventeenth century, just over 150 medical texts had been published in English; half a century later, more than 200 were published within a twenty-year period alone.[9] This explosion of medical book publishing did include books of learned and philosophical bio-medicine such as Crooke's, but the greater number were intended for practical use in the home. Almanacs, books of remedies, treatises on the diagnosis and treatment of particular diseases such as the plague and the pox, and, increasingly, books on women's healthcare filled the literary marketplace and served a population of literate but unlatined middling and upper-class men and women. Many of these books were cheap and physically small, printed in quartos and octavos more often than in folios, and their stated intention was to offer basic instruction in the details of medical diagnosis and the options and techniques for medical treatment. The books on women's healthcare sometimes included cursory treatments of issues typical of a more philosophical bio-medicine such as the constitutional causes of sterility or the physiological process of conception, but the emphasis consistently was on diagnosis and therapy more than on the theoretical aspects of medicine. They offered advice on how to identify and manage diseases and conditions particular to women (such as "womb fury" and "green sickness"), and instruction on issues relating to pregnancy, delivery, and, frequently, nursing and childcare. By and large these were derivative texts, translations and compilations of Continental sources and older English medical material. They catered to a medical culture in which self-diagnosis and self-treatment were normative, and they included both those that claimed to replace professional practitioners (like Sudell's) and those that proposed more simply to aid in a patient's dealing with a professional practitioner, be that a physician, as Sadler's text does, or a midwife. Though their commercial motivations are rarely hidden—some of the texts even advertise the specific apothecaries who sell their authors' unique remedies—these books form an integral part of the widespread vernacular popularization of medicine in the sixteenth and seventeenth centuries.[10]

As practical advice books and guides to bio-medical self-help, these books differ from Crooke's learned and philosophical bio-medicine in both genre and audience. Focused on practical instructions for diagnosis and treatment, they are essentially how-to manuals; as a group, they therefore typically assume an audience not of elite and bookish men, but of women as well as men, professional practitioners and lay people alike, intent on acting on the practical advice offered.

These differences in genre and audience are significant to the patterns of the self deployed in the healthcare manuals, for instructional manuals and their implied audience of actors necessitate a model of personhood not unlike the one that characterizes Crooke's normative man—an agent able to act purposively on a conceptually separable body. These manuals always assume volitional, coherent persons who are encouraged to care for their own and others' bodies; sometimes these persons take the form of characters in the text itself, as in James Wolveridge's *Speculum matricis hybernicum*, in which a physician tests the proficiency of a fictional midwife's knowledge of her craft in a question-and-answer format.[11] More commonly, an agential reader emerges through repeated grammatical formulations, through the imperative, for example, which implies the second person ("If [the flux] proceeds from crudities in the stomacke . . . take every morning of the decoction of lignum sanctum"),[12] or through the jussive, which implies the third person (if the menses have stopped, "Let the Patient so grieved, sweat; for that opens the Pores."[13] A reader thus constructed might be told how to tailor her diet to promote fertility, how to distinguish between a true and false conception, or how to treat a certain windiness of the womb. Volitional subjectivity is routinely assumed in these texts but specifically as a rhetorical function of their genre.

It is important to recognize the relation between the agential subject and the genre of instructional manuals precisely because the promise of female person-hood proffered by the genre does not correlate with the medical conception of women in these texts. Though they envision an audience of self-determining actors, these manuals as a group never align the physiological female with the characteristics of emerging personhood—disembodied agency, for example, or stable autonomy. Despite their typically confident tone, with authors present-ing themselves as possessed of the best, most reliable medical advice, the texts are suffused with tensions and anxieties about the content, meanings, and uses of medical knowledge; considered cumulatively, and especially in the therapeutics the texts promote, these instabilities ultimately make impossible female partic-ipation in the emerging (male) model of personhood.

■ That agential subjectivity is an aspect of the genre more than a register of the medically conceived female is neatly demonstrated by the one text that most exclusively *is* an instructional manual, the first edition of *The Byrth of Mankynde*.[14] *The Byrth of Mankynde* was both the first book on gynecology and obstetrics printed in English and the one most frequently reprinted through the first half of the seventeenth century; it went through at least fourteen editions between 1540 and 1654 and continued to be reissued until 1676. The 1540 edition is Richard Jonas's translation of *De partu hominis* (1532), which is itself a Latin translation of a Ger-man text written in 1513. That text in turn, written by Eucharius Rösslin, was based on a late-medieval manuscript of a sixth-century version of a second-century work on gynecology attributed to Soranus. The medical material in these books is thus mostly derivative and quite ancient. Books I and II of the 1540 edition contain Jonas's fairly literal translation of Rösslin, treating the positions of the fetus in the womb and instructions for handling a birth, along with a discussion of the diseases of and care for children "lately born"; Book III, Jonas's addition, treats the question of conception and the problem of sterility. The book also con-tains copperplate engravings depicting possible fetal positions that derive at least from the eleventh century, along with engravings of reproductive anatomy derived from Vesalius.[15]

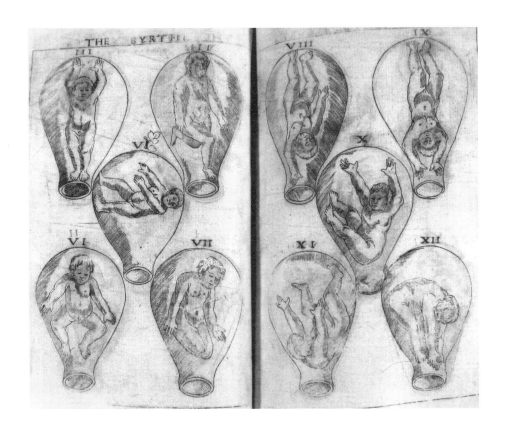

*Plate 4. From Richard Jonas,* The Byrth of Mankynde *(London, 1540), the plate depicts positions of the fetus in the womb. Reproduced by permission of the New York Academy of Medicine Library.*

Unlike most of the other books of its kind in English, Jonas's 1540 version of *The Byrth of Mankynde* is exclusively practical in its presentation and straightforward in its advice; in its clear-cut, unreflective recommendations, it conceives of the childbearing woman *solely* in the agential mode of an instructional manual. Concerned neither with the arcane causes of medical problems nor with wider physiological or cosmological congruencies into which practical medical knowledge fits, the book provides conventional information on the process of labor and delivery, the more and less common difficulties that attend them, and sketchy counsel on how to handle them. It includes numerous recipes for perfumes and pills, "clisters, odors, and oyntements," for treating all issues related to childbearing and birth, from making labor easier to provoking the birth and restraining the flux of blood afterwards.

Although the ordeal of labor and delivery is repeatedly described as being fraught with danger and the childbearing woman as threatened with possible death in addition to certain pain, the woman is nonetheless portrayed as being fully, actively, and verbally a participant in her labor and the delivery. It is she, for example, who determines when labor is imminent:

> [W]hen the woman perceaveth the matrice or mother to wax laxe or loose and to be dissolved and that the humours yssue forthe in greate plente then shall it be mete for her to syt downe lenynge backwarde in manner upryght. (*J.BM*, XX v)

In an age before the entrance of men into the birthing room, before what has been called the medicalization of childbirth, *Byrth* unproblematically assumes that the parturient woman can "perceave" her body and its internal workings: she can perceive not only what is apparent *outside* her body, the issuing of humors "in great plente," but what's *inside*, too, the matrix waxing loose. Without having to rely on another's assessment of her condition, the woman herself determines the time to sit down and prepare for the birth. Similarly, though a birthing chair is recommended as providing the best position for delivery (and the book includes an engraving of a birthing stool), the woman herself is assumed to be able to determine what is the best position for her, whatever "shall seme commodious and necessarye to the partie" (*J.BM*, XXV v). And the author recognizes that the best circumstance for delivery generally is when "the woman is stronge and myghtye of nature and such as can well and strongelye helpe her self to the expellynge of the byrth" (*J.BM*, XVII r). Though the child, too, is assumed to help in its own delivery, the parturient woman "her selfe" expels the birth.

The parturient woman is thus portrayed as a self-knowing, volitional agent, beset by peril but assumed able to acquire aid when necessary. The author urges women to be not ashamed or abashed if their delivery becomes difficult but rather to "disclose theyr mynde" to the called-in physician and show him everything "so that the phisition understandynge the womans mynde maye the soner by his learnynge and experience consyder the true cause of it and the very remedy to amend it" (*J.BM*, XXXV v). Not silent before the authority of the physician, the parturient woman is construed as a necessary agent in her own health. The book is not intended to replace the need for a physician but it does assume that the woman will contribute to managing her own care.

The unproblematized agency of the parturient woman in Jonas's translation of *Byrth* is perhaps most neatly expressed in its revision of the traditional understanding of the pain of childbirth. Labor and delivery always entail suffering, and the myriad imagined possibilities for added distress—from a "narrow passage" or "emerrodes" (hemorrhoids) to a fetus presenting feet-first or, worse, one that comes forth with "two heddes" (*J.BM*, XIIII v–XV r)—are recognized to cause the woman to sustain "greate douloure payne and anguyshe" (*J.BM*, XV r). But if Jonas emphasizes the perils and pain women must (passively) suffer, as most such texts do, he nevertheless reconfigures the experience of pain and thereby implicitly what it signifies about women's nature. Traditionally, the pain of childbirth was understood to be the fulfillment of God's curse on Eve for her disobedience in Eden; pain was normative and the mark of divine displeasure. Though empathy with the suffering woman was not thereby restricted, a woman's pain was yet another proof of the female's inherent imperfection. On the verso of the title page of his translation of *Byrth*, however, Jonas, while remembering the Biblical associations of childbirth pain, realigns their meaning. His intent, he says, in making the book available in English is to aid

> the women whiche systayne and endure for the tyme so greate dolor and payne for the byrth of Mankyndee and delyueraunce of the same in to the worlde. (*J.BM*, t.p. v)

Women suffer pain for a purpose, not passively as a sign of sin but actively as a means to deliver mankind. In this act of willful self-sacrifice, enduring dolor for the sake of deliverance, women act not in the stain of Eve but in imitation of Christ, who suffered to save the world.

The first printing of the first book on childbirth in English, taken up as it mostly is with unelaborated instruction, constructs the parturient woman as an agent able to manage her body. To whatever extent somatic experience is considered to be meaningful, it signifies in ways that endorse this sense of the childbearing woman as fully participatory in, and thereby conceptually separable from, her bodily life. One could, then, on the basis of this single text, make the case that the female, as medically constructed in the gynecological literature of the period, *did* participate in the emerging ideal of the early modern individual. Here, both the implied reader and the described patient are self-aware, self-directing, and treated as entities separate from but able to act on their bodies. And because Jonas's edition of *Byrth* has no theoretical asides, no disquisitions on the meaning of medical knowledge, no labored justifications for making that knowledge widely available to the reading public, there is nothing in the text to counter the individuated, volitional self that exists in the text as a genre-based characteristic of instructional manuals.

But this unreflective presentation of medical material is actually anomalous in the period. Though almanacs and books on medical recipes typically did proceed by way of simple lists, books on women's healthcare more frequently included at least some interpretive glossing of medical practice, some evaluative analysis of medical knowledge. In these texts, more common and more prolix, other understandings of the female emerge, and typically in contexts fraught with anxiety about what femaleness is, who gets to know about it, and what readers might do with the knowledge.

A new edition of *Byrth* was published five years after its first appearance; in 1545, Thomas Raynalde, claiming to find the earlier translation of Rösslin by a "studious and dilygent clarke" (Jonas) too literal, had a corrected and emended edition of the text printed. To the pragmatic, treatment-oriented material drawn from Rösslin and Jonas, Raynalde added an entire book on Galenic reproductive anatomy, a chapter on cosmetics, and a long prologue justifying his additions (*R.BM*, Bi v–Bii r). Although the cosmetic material is equally as unelaborated as the material from Rösslin, the chapter on anatomy and the long preface are considerably more expansive. These two new sections (which became standard in all subsequent editions of the book) demonstrate a new note of anxiety concerning medical learning about women. In addition to the practical information contained in Jonas's edition, Raynalde retains the clear sense of the woman as a participatory patient, an intelligent actor in the labor of healthcare, but in the process of contemplating the information he offers, Raynalde reveals its many vexations.

Raynalde begins his new translation with a defense of anatomy. He argues that one cannot understand the practice of physic without first knowing something of its foundation in anatomy; happily, however, this knowledge is readily attainable because anatomy itself is certain. Anatomy, he says, is the basis for all the "wittinesse and artificiall crafty inuention" of the noble science of physic (*R.BM*, Biiii v). It is

> the foundation and ground, by the perceaveraunce wherof your wittes and under-standing shall be illuminat and lyghtnyd, the better to understand, how euery thyng cumeth to passe within your bodyes in tyme of conception, of baryng, and of byrth. (*R.BM*, Biii v)

Anatomy will teach how everything comes to pass; the argument, rather extravagant perhaps but good for marketing, is that "every thyng" having to do with "the byrth of mankynde"—the processes of conception, bearing, and birth—are not only fully *knowable* through anatomy, but are in fact *already known*. Furthermore, Raynalde suggests that with this full and certain knowledge clearly in her possession, a woman will be able to act in partnership with her physician should something go awry:

> For note ye well, that as there is no man what euer he be that shall become an abso-lut and perfeict phisition onles he have an absolut and perfeict knowledge of all the inwardes and outwardes of mans and womans body. . . . Agayn when that a woman cometh to a phisition for conceil, concerning sume thing that may be amysse in that part: the answere of the phisition and reasonable allegation of causes to the same infirmyte is many tymes obscure, darke, and straunge, to be comprehended by the woman for lacke of due knowledge of the situationn, maner, and facion of the inwards. (*R.BM*, Biii v–Biiii r)

As in Jonas's edition, the woman here is conceived as an intellectually capable participant in healthcare. Though she is not explicitly advised to dispense with a physician, she is assumed to be able to understand and therefore to comply with a physician's counsel.

Raynalde's argument is built on a confidence both in medical knowledge itself and in its deployment by resourceful women who will read his material for their own betterment. But this seeming stability of knowledge and its deployment becomes precarious as soon as Raynalde reflects on who his readers might be and how they might interpret his words. The women he addresses here are not only childbearing women, as in Jonas's version; Raynalde's edition is addressed to women readers generally and he explicitly urges "all women" to strive to understand what he teaches. This sense of an enlarged audience of women defined more by social condition than by professional affiliation is also suggested by his inclusion of the material on cosmetics, which, he says, is intended to help honorable women "obtayne the loue, amitie, and harty perpetuall fauour fyrst of God, and then of all honest, discrete, and godly wyse men" (*R.BM*, vii r).

Raynalde's audience is thus rather large—a middling class of women, probably but not necessarily literate (since he says that he has heard of women reading the book to others), and able to afford both cosmetics and the medicines made by the advertised apothecaries. But the very openness of the audience raises concerns about how it will interpret his work, how all his advice will be taken. This nervousness is to some extent a conventional trope of books about women's health, particularly those about reproduction.[16] But here the anxiety is both heightened and elaborated; whereas Jonas, for example, has a one-page "admonition to the reader" in which he succinctly and predictably expresses his hope that readers will use the proffered information for the benefit of women rather than any purpose bawdy or lewd, Raynalde develops this conventional concern into a broader and more fretful discussion of the volatility of interpretation.

Even if all the nine muses graced his work, Raynalde reflects, still there would be those who would deride it, either because they would still consider it unseemly to speak plainly of women's matters in our mother tongue or because, by learning the "secrets" of women, they would be moved "to abhorre and loothe the company of woomen" (*R.BM*, Cii r); there is something shameful about medical knowledge of women or something so awful inherent to it that readers will eschew women altogether. But Raynalde realizes that he has no control over his audience; men will read the book as much as women, and though he encourages women to not mind their husbands reading "such thynges"—"for many men there be of so gentyll and louynge nature towards theyr wyfes, that they wyll be moore diligent and carefull to reade or seke out any thing that shold do theyr wyfes gud being in that case then the wemen them selues" (*R.BM*, Cvii r–v)—he knows full well that the book is equally available to "every boy and knave" who will enjoy it "as openly as the tales of Robine hood" (*R.BM*, D v). Written as a medical self-help guide for women, the book can just as easily become an entertainment for boys.

Recognizing what is beyond his control and anxious about its implications, Raynalde seeks a solution by reconceiving the meaning of medical knowledge and repositioning the origin of its interpretation. The problem, he proposes, lies not with the information but with the readers, who determine the value of information solely by how they choose to use it. There is nothing so pure, he says, not fire or water, not Scripture or even the Sacrament, that it cannot be abused; but "to them that be goud themselves, euerye thing turnith to goud" (*R.BM*, Ciiii v). Value lies solely in the reader, not in what is read. Therefore, he reasons,

> Consyderyng that there is nothyng in this world so necessary, ne so goud, holy or vertuouse, but that it may by wickednysse be abused, it shall be no great wunder though this lytel booke also, made, written, and set furth for a good pourpose, yet by lyght and lewde persons be used contrary to godlynesse, honesty, or th'entent of the wryter there of. (*R.BM*, Ciiii v)

Raynalde insists on the meaning he wants to convey: there is nothing "in woman so priyve ne so secret that they shold nede to care who knew of it"; neither is there "any part in woman moore to be abhorred then in man" (*R.BM*, Cvi r–v). But the very vigor of his argument belies his anxiety about its efficacy. Value, he has told us, lies in the reader—it cannot be controlled by assertions of authorial intent—but however good or godly his own intent, Raynalde knows very well that "lewd, unhappy, and knavish" people may very well read the book (*R.BM*, Cvi v).

Raynalde's preface thus founders on an opposition. It promises an impossible certainty of knowledge but immediately thereafter demonstrates a concern precisely about the certainty of its use. Raynalde claims that readers will understand "how every thing cumeth to passe within [their] bodyes" (*R.BM*, Biii v) but then he frets over how that knowledge might be understood. This tension, between knowledge about women's bodies and its manifold meanings, is characteristic of Raynalde's added material, and it plays out as well in his added chapter on reproductive anatomy. Here, Raynalde follows fairly traditional Galenism, incorporating both anatomical and physiological details that he treats as uncontested. But even as he does so, he seems to struggle with their implications, with what they might suggest about women's nature and about the assumed hierarchy between women and men.

For example, Raynalde treats the womb as any Galenic physiologist would. Endowed with the natural faculties of attraction, retention, alteration, and expulsion, the womb acts in a typically subjectified way. The womb port, he says, does "naturally open it selfe, attractynge, drawing, and suckyng into the wombe the seede by a vehement and naturall desyre" (*R.BM*, 14r). And the womb itself, called "the mother," acts like a good mother as it contracts around the conception:

[I]n tyme of conception of the seede, the lytell bolke or quantite of the sayd seede at this fyrste conceyuyng into the womans mother may be toochyd round about every where of the mother: and as ye wold say amplexd or embraced and containyd. (*R.BM*, 11r–v)

But even as Raynalde incorporates conventionally subjectified Galenic body parts and describes their intentional functioning in traditionally Galenic ways, imputing maternal nurturance to the contractions of the womb, in this instance, he does not as routinely accept the equally conventional meanings associated with Galenic physiology. This is particularly the case in his discussion of the normative two-seed model of conception, when he comes up against the traditional understanding of the homology. Because women and men have the same generative parts, differing essentially in their placement, both are understood to emit seed during copulation, and it is the combined seed of the male and the female that constitutes the conception.[17] In explaining this process of conception, Raynalde takes recourse in its standard qualification: both male and female have seed, but "the seede and sparme" of woman is emphatically not as "stronge, ferme, and mighty in operation as the seede of man"; it is, rather, "weke, fluy, cold, and moyst, and of no grete fyrmitie" (*R.BM*, 14 v–15 r). He endorses this Galenic truism and yet, some ten pages later, he begins to equivocate, as if to recalibrate his scale of value, when he repeats the seemingly self-evident, that there is "nothing so firme, perfect, absolut, and myghty in woma[n] as in man":

Yet you can not cal this any imperfection or lacke in woman: for the woman in her kynd, and for the office and pourpose where for she was made, is even as absolute and perfect as man in his kynd; nether is woman to be callyd (as sum do) unperfecter then man, (for bycause that man is moore myghtyer and strong: the woman wekar, more feble). (*R.BM*, 24 r)

A "geldyd" man is imperfect in comparison to other men, Raynalde explains, but a woman is not imperfect in comparison to man because the medical homology breaks down at the point of its meaning—woman is not of the same kind as man, and valuation is telling only *within* kinds, not *across* them. This is a significant divergence from Galen, for whom woman was precisely an incomplete man, an embodiment of lack conceivable only in relation to man. For Galen, this imperfection, this lack, is teleologically purposive and entirely for the best, for without this imperfection in woman, reproduction would be impossible, but woman nonetheless has no positive existence separate from her position relative to man.[18] Raynalde, it seems, accepts the Galenic medical model, the basic isomorphism between male and female generative products, but revises its standard associations for gender difference. One may read Raynalde's revision as either better or worse for women; since, according to Raynalde's preface, value lies in the reader anyway, one could argue about whether the more positive picture of sex relations emerges from the model of woman as different in kind from man or as a lesser version of man. But however one values the revision, it is important to note that it *is* a revision, that Raynalde is at least implicitly aware that medical knowledge, seemingly so certain, has the potential for multiple meanings. Raynalde's opening promise, therefore, of certain knowledge and clear instruction on "how a woman with childe shal use her selfe" founders on the evidence of the text itself, which traffics in uncertainty and anxiety about the variable possible meanings and uses of medical knowledge about women.

Raynalde's edition of *The Byrth of Mankynde* was the most commonly reprinted book on childbearing and childbirth up to the mid-seventeenth century. Though it continued to be printed in new editions until 1676, its popularity was superceded after 1651, when Nicholas Culpeper published *A Directory for Midwives*, which became the most often reprinted manual of its kind through the end of the seventeenth century.[19] Written just over 100 years after Raynalde's edition of *Byrth*, *A Directory for Midwives* shows a significant shift in the meanings of medical knowledge about women. Though it is still thoroughly based in Galenic anatomy and physiology, *A Directory for Midwives* is repeatedly and explicitly ready to admit both Galen's errors and the extent of current controversy about matters biomedical. And yet the significant shift in the century that separates Culpeper from Raynalde inheres less in the increasing skepticism about the ancient renditions of the body, for these questionings and doubts are easily apparent and explicitly addressed by Culpeper himself. What is more telling is how certain Culpeper is about the *meanings* of the female body, even as the *models* for understanding the body are so explicitly open to question. As much as Culpeper admits the breadth of factual uncertainty, he is all the more adamant about the body's meanings. And the meanings that he is sure of make impossible any stable sense of a volitional, agential woman.

Nicholas Culpeper, who called himself "a student in astrology and physic," was the most prolific popularizer of medical learning in seventeenth-century England.[20] He wrote vehemently against what he saw as the monopolistic abuses of the College of Physicians, repeatedly charging its practitioners with a self-interested disregard for both the poor and the dangerously ill. A political radical as much as an advocate for medical reform, Culpeper, an Independent with Leveller sympathies, fought against the King during the Civil War. After being shot in the chest at the battle of Newberry in 1643, he retired to the countryside where, under the auspices of the printer Peter Cole, he set about translating noted contemporary medical texts from Latin. Over the next decade or so, until his death in 1654, he translated enough material for Cole to advertise the collection as *The Rational Physicians Library*, which included, among many others, a translation of the fiercely protected *Pharmacopoeia Londinenisis* of the College of Physicians.[21] This was the College's authoritative text on pharmacology; it included all the remedies the College approved of and was intended to be used only by the apothecaries who prepared the medicines their physicians prescribed. Culpeper's translating of the *Pharmacopoeia* into English defied established medical authority as much as his taking up the Parliamentarian cause defied the authority of the King. The preface to his translation, published in 1649, makes the connection clear: "The Prize which We now . . . play for, is, THE LIBERTY OF THE SUBJECT."[22] Just as war abolished tyrannical authority in the state, so might translations like his abolish tyrannical authority in medicine, and the *subject* would be free.

Culpeper continues in his reformist zeal in *A Directory for Midwives*, published in 1651. His overall intent, he says, is to make available to English readers everything they need to know about "the preservation of Man, even from his cradle to his grave" (*DM*, A4r). Though his monetary interests are never really disguised— for fuller treatments of the topic at hand he routinely refers readers to other books he has produced—there is a pervasive sense in all his books that his mission is charitable at least as much as it is financial, and that his intent is to make medical learning and practice as widely available as possible. In *Directory*, he even expresses a self-deprecating though perhaps not wholehearted humility; though his desire is to instruct midwives in the bases and rudiments of their craft, he recognizes their superior practical experience in the birthing room, and so he opens himself willingly to their "emendation" (ibid.).[23]

As a reformer, as a ready iconoclast, Culpeper is not at all blindly bound to Galenic tradition , even as be brings to light Galenic bio-medicine about the childbearing body. He echoes the common complaint that Galen "never saw a Man nor Woman dissected in his life time" (*DM*, 27), attributing Galen's mistakes, such as supposing the womb to have multiple cavities rather than one, to his inexperience in human anatomy (*DM*, 23). And he recognizes, too, that much about generation is not known, or he claims it simply irrelevant to the practice of medicine. How precisely the fetus is formed in the womb, whether women have seed as well as men, whether hermaphrodites really exist—these are all traditional questions that Culpeper considers "trifles" in the disputes between the Ancients and the Moderns (*DM*, 53).

But for all his modern willingness to critique Galen and to see biophilosophical questions as unrelated to practical physic, the body for Culpeper is still basically Galenic, both in terms of anatomy and physiology and in the sense of its seamless connection to the rest of the natural world. For Culpeper, as much as for Crooke, man is to be understood as the epitome of creation, housing within him the principles and powers that pervade the cosmos. As in *Microcosmographia*, the body in *Directory* is replete with meaning, and knowledge of its structures and processes teaches not only medical lessons about maintaining health and curing disease but moral lessons about human life as well. If Raynalde, 100 years earlier, struggled with the open-endedness of those lessons, Culpeper by contrast, in his religious and medical zeal, refuses to entertain such ambiguity.

As a teacher of the body's lessons, making available in the vernacular what has previously been held secret, Culpeper treats his medical writing as an aspect of salvific history, a liberation patterned on divine interventions in time. God himself, he explains, has appointed the office of the midwife, and it is to Him that midwives ultimately will have to give account for their work (*DM*, 6). Culpeper therefore characterizes the lack of available knowledge as the product of an enslavement comparable to the bondage of the Israelites in Egypt (*DM*, A5r), and his attempt to liberate knowledge from the covetous clutches of learned physicians as analogous to Moses's wresting the Hebrews from the Pharaoh's unhealthy embrace. In another version of the same idea, the crabbed and difficult sounding physicians are likened to the Rabbis in the days of Christ, who "muffle up our Eyes" with "strange Names" lest we should "see the Truth" (*DM*, 7). Given his religious and political commitments, however, he most commonly tropes the physicians as Papists, money-hungry, self-interested, and concerned more for their own authority than for the welfare of those they pretend to serve:

My Country Men and Women, who have been two [sic] long reined in with the bridle of Ignorance by Physitians, that so they might the better be ridden by them, for just for all the world as the Popish Priests serve those they cal the Laity . . . so do our Physitians serve the commonalty of this Nation: viz. Hide all from them they can, for they know . . . that should the vulgar but be a little acquainted with their

Mysteries, all their jugling and knavery would be seen, and their wealth and esteem, which is the Diana they adore, would be put to a non-plus. (*DM*, 17–18)

Despite his modern protestations about the value of observations (he has seen human dissections, whereas Galen has not) in the context of such a typological view of providential history, human truths are not extrapolated from the body but are rather demonstrated by it. The neck of the womb, what we would call the vaginal canal, for example, is "seated between the passage of Urine and the right gut to show proud man what little reason he hath to be proud and domineer[ing], being conceived between the places ordained to cast out excrements, the very sinks of the Body, and in such a manner that his Mother was ashamed to tell him how"( *DM*, 25). The placement of the neck of the womb is purposive, not so much in terms of physiology as in terms of moral meaning; it sits between the places of excrement to teach a lesson in humility.

If some of the lessons Culpeper expounds are explicit, such as the one taught by the placement of the neck of the womb or by the womb's ability to expand and contract, which "gives cause to every one of us" he says, "to admire at the wonderful Works of God in the Creation of Man" (*DM*, 26), others are less obviously drawn. Yet these, too, maintain an a priori certainty even in the face of admittedly contested knowledge. Discussing, for example, whether or not hymens exist, a topic currently of "much controversie amongst Anatomists" (*DM*, 23), Culpeper finds it particularly troublesome that its presence or absence is used as a sign of virginity. He is willing to withhold judgment on the anatomical evidence but he cannot doubt the a priori truth of Scripture, and it is this more than the anatomists' debate that determines what to learn from the body's ambiguities. Noting that "God gave to the Hebrews" this "note of Virginity," Culpeper claims that "it is naturally in all Virgins, unless they break it with their fingers . . . For it is no way probable, that God would have given that for a certain sign of virginity, which Columbus and Ambros Pary say is not alwaies found . . . it is very probable the Hebrew Virgins were more chary in preserving it, than the Italians were" (*DM*, 24). The anatomy may be controversial but the questionable moral character of the Italians is not.

A similar tension between pre-established meaning and contested information occurs even more tellingly in Culpeper's use of the Galenic homology between male and female generative parts. He employs the homology in describing the female anatomy, but it seems in his hands less a means to assert a purported similarity than to delineate a fundamental difference. Having already discussed the stones in men ("called in Latin, Testes, that is, Witness, because they witness one to be a Man") (*DM*, 11), Culpeper introduces the corresponding chapter on women simply as follows:

The Stones of Women (for they have such kind of toys as wel as Men) differ from the Stones of Men. (*DM*, 29)

That women as well as men have stones is for Culpeper an explanatory problem: if stones, or testes, witness one to be a *man*, the anatomical evidence that women have "such kind of toys as wel as Men" must be overridden by some prewritten meaning. The seeming similarity conveyed by the name points in truth to hierarchical difference. The nine points of difference he lists, in place, magnitude, form, figure, substance, are unambiguously valued; women's stones are "less," "uneven," "not stayed" and "depressed" compared to men's. Even the differences that do not seem weighted in this way get absorbed nonetheless in the hierarchy. That women's stones are "within," for example, is accepted unquestioningly as an aspect of women's relative weakness, a symptom of their colder, read inferior, temperature. There is never for Culpeper any question of why cold, for example, should be regarded as inferior or why the marks of difference need to be understood hierarchically at all. These are givens for him, predetermined truths that remain even as the medical models that purport to demonstrate them are increasingly opened to question.

Though a revolutionary against traditional medical authority and aware of contemporary debate about matters both anatomical and physiological, Culpeper's appropriation of conventional meanings is nonetheless more unbending, more thoroughly entrenched than Raynalde's 100 years earlier. Even as the medical models begin to waver, if only slightly, their associated meanings grow firmer. Dismissing as irrelevant the instability of its ancient models, the body becomes for him the bedrock on which to ground the a priori and unequivocal truths of gender hierarchy.

Culpeper's certainty about the relative inferiority of females makes it impossible for him to write an autonomous female subjectivity in any sustained way. As a book of practical physic, *Directory* does incorporate the language of agential action—the rhetoric assumes an individual, for example, who can accurately regulate her diet so that she consumes exactly as much as her stomach can concoct; this way the food will be transformed purely to nourishing blood without overmuch "crudity," and this in turn will help to ensure healthy conceptions because they will be generated from healthful seed made of healthful blood (*DM*, 34f). But at same time as he writes of an idealized autonomous agent who knows exactly how much food her body needs, Culpeper equally engages typical Galenic rhetoric of personified parts. Thus a healthy womb embraces and cherishes the seed and, when wounded by scarring or ulceration, it becomes barren, more concerned to "succour itself . . . [like] a Man that is sick or wounded" than to take care of its proper "business" of conceiving (*DM*, 27).

These two alternate, vying modes of agency, possessed by an implied person and a body part, however, ultimately get absorbed in another, more pervasive, model, in which both the person and the part, the woman and the womb, together become the instrument (the organ) of a higher autonomy. In the chapter in which he discusses the "Formation of the Child in the Womb," Culpeper offers a roughly Galenic primer on embryogenesis. He admits that this is "the difficultest piece of work in the whole book" because it is so rare to see a pregnant woman opened (*DM*, 48). He, however, has seen "a Woman opened that died in Child-bed, not delivered," and yet the majority of the discussion focuses not on what he saw but on what can only be speculated about—the earliest stages of embryogenesis and fetal development. And despite his repeated reservations about Galen, who "never saw a Man nor Woman dissected in his life time" (*DM*, 27), the theory of embryogenesis is thoroughly Galenic: "in the act of copulation, the Woman spends her Seed as wel as the Man, and both are united to make the Conception" (*DM*, 48). That is the basic idea, and the details are Galenic, too; for example, the idea that the sex of the child is determined by whether the man's or the woman's seed is stronger (*DM*, 49) and the idea that the liver is formed before the heart (*DM*, 50). But tellingly absent from his description is a Galenic, agential womb. The womb is not here described as acting with the inherent faculties it is said elsewhere to possess. Womb and woman act as non-volitional agents of a higher-order Nature in the creation of the fetus. As soon as conception occurs from the mixing of the two seeds, Culpeper explains,

> the first thing which is operative in the Conception is the spirit, whereof the seed is ful; this Spirit Nature quickeneth by the heat of the Womb, and stirs it up to action. (*DM*, 49)

Nature quickens the spirit *by* the heat of the womb; it is Nature that fashions the fetus, using the womb as its instrument. A little later Culpeper directly raises the question, "whether the active power of forming lie in the womb, or not"

(*DM*, 53), but he considers this, as well as other questions regarding the conception (such as whether the seed is the "efficient cause of our formation" or whether the seed "flow from all parts of the body") to be ultimately "frivolous" and "needless Disputes" (ibid.). Although he does not answer any of these questions directly, his rhetoric suggests his assumption that although active power is carried out *by* the womb, that power is not *in* or *of* it.

The difference from Galen is subtler here than it was in Raynalde's treatment of the homology of generative parts, but it is not thereby less telling. For Galen, as for Culpeper here, Nature can be rendered as the supreme agent in conception, and persons, both male and female, can be considered the instruments by which she enacts her purposive patterns. But in Galen, persons are conceived of as inseparable from Nature, as aspects of her, and Nature herself is both and equally transcendent and immanent in individuals. In Culpeper, by contrast, Nature's agency is conceived of *in contrast to* the individual's; it is Nature's agency, not the woman's or the womb's, that quickens the spirit.

This opposition between women's and Nature's agency is even more starkly apparent in the sections on the longings of women with child. Here, Culpeper explains that these pangs of desire arise when women are immoderate in the so-called non-naturals, things such as meat and drink, sleep and watching, exercise and rest (*DM*, 119). When this occurs, when women choose to act against nature, Nature intervenes to correct the imbalance:

> Nature [is] the chief Artificer, [and] calls for such food as must make fitting blood for the Nourishment, or encrease of the Child; your child is nourished by your blood, your blood is bred by your diet, rectified or marred by your exercise, idleness, sleep, or watching; etc. Nature sees and knows how you swerve from what is fitting, she calls, and calls like a Work woman for what is requisite either to make up what you want, or to remedy what you have done amiss, by breeding a nourishment for the child within you contrary to what diet or things not natural you have formerly kept. (*DM*, 120)

Here Culpeper envisions a fully agential individual who is simultaneously subject to the greater agential power of Nature, which has the ability to induce longings in women. Women may experience the longings as theirs, as aspects of their own somatic will, but what seems to be of the individual is reconceived as having been in fact implanted in the individual by Nature, acting to protect the fetus against the bad behaviors of the woman.

Having absorbed the quickening of the spirit and the longings of the woman into the higher purposes of Nature, Culpeper concludes his consideration on the formation of the child by relegating miscarriage, too, to Nature's design:

> I have done, only take notice, that Nature not having her desire (and she desires nothing but what is needful, perhaps of necessity) is forced to let go the Conception for want of necessaries, and then the women miscarries and who can blame her? The children of Israel could not make bricks if they had not straw. (*DM*, 121)

When women willfully deny Nature her desires by not properly caring for themselves when with child, Nature blamelessly lets go the conception. Like the children of Israel, bound and abused by an oppressive taskmaster, Nature is held captive, for a time, by a willful woman. The image of Culpeper's preface returns, only here it is Nature, not knowledge, that is bound, and women are not the gladdened recipients of Culpeper's salvific liberation but the foolhardy perpetrators of an unintended destruction.

If *Directory* offers variable models for understanding women's anatomy and physiology, it seems less variable and eclectic than Galenic thought in its assumptions about what that medical knowledge means, particularly about how woman, medically conceived, stands, by herself and in relation to man. Galenic tradition might err, both in theoretical and practical physic, but the cultural configurations with which it has typically been allied do not. For Culpeper, much more so than for the editors of *The Byrth of Mankynde*, woman has little existence in her own right; she is construed either as a lesser version of man, an instance of absence, or as an instrument of a higher agency that occludes any stable sense of her own being.

■ The troubled condition of medical knowledge about women may also be profitably explored among the diagnoses and recommended therapies for womb-related ailments, the single cause, as Sadler suggested, of woman's grief. For here the uneasy connection between person and part, woman and womb, is most apparent. Advice about the diagnosis and treatment of women's diseases typically conflates descriptions of persons suffering from some manner of disease with more insistently described demands of a desirous and rebellious womb. Part of the rhetorical confusion that besets these therapies results from the persistent though long denied notion of the womb as itself an animal, wracked by desires and wandering around the body wreaking havoc unless it is satisfied. But even when all writers were easily disavowing that belief, recognizing, as even Galen had, that the womb was held in place by ligaments and could not wander as an independently-willed animal, many therapeutic interventions for womb-related diseases still managed to treat the womb as the predominant agent of female existence.[24]

One example of this pattern is the description and recommended treatment for an ailment called "madness of the womb." In a work translated from Latin by Culpeper, Lazarus Riverius explains that womb fury

> is a sort of Madness arising from a vehement unbridled desire of Carnal Imbracement, which desire dis-thrones the Rational Faculty so far, that the Patient utters wanton and lascivious Speeches, in all places and companies; and having cast off all modesty, madly seeks after Carnal Copulation, and invites men to have to do with her in that way.[25]

Riverius here portrays a fully delineated woman and not just a womb, a patient uttering wanton and lascivious speeches, madly seeking sex. It is clear that the problem to be treated is unbridled desire, but this initial description of the disease does not say where precisely the desire resides—whether its seat is in the woman as a whole, as a person whose rational faculty has been dethroned and who is therefore driven by the irresistible imperatives of appetite, or whether it lies more specifically in her womb. So Riverius clarifies by way of explaining cause:

> This Immoderate desire of Carnal Conjunction, springs from the abundance of Seed, from its Acrimony, and heat transcending the bounds of Nature, whereby it is made to heave and work in the Seminal vessels as Yest [sic] works, whereby the parts made for generation, are vehemently stirred up, and Inflamed with lustful desires. (*PP*, 417–18)

In standard Galenic fashion, womb fury arises when an abundance of seed accumulates and then foments in the womb, overheats, and stirs up lust in the parts made for generation. Thus the name of the disease has a double significance; it indicates a woman's fury (caused by the womb) and also the fury of the womb itself. The woman wanders crazed, but it is the womb that suffers from lustful desire. One way to treat this dual disorder is to try to cool the overheated womb and this is done by bloodletting, balms, or diets that decrease body temperature.

But since the initial problem arises from an accumulation of unreleased seed, the most effective cure is simply to provide a means for getting rid of it:

> In regard of the immediate Cause, seeing the evacuating of the sharp and corrupted Seed, may cure the Disease; it is very good Advice in the beginning of the Disease, before the Patient begins manifestly to rave, or in the space between her fits, when she is pretty well, to marry her to a lusty young man. For so the Womb being satisfied, and the offensive Matter contained in its Vessels being emptied, the Patient may peradventure be cured. (*PP*, 419)

It seems for Riverius, then, in the disease called madness of the womb, that though it is the woman who utters wanton speech, it is the womb that needs sex because it is the womb and not the woman per se that will be "satisfied" by marriage to "a lusty young man." A description that begins with a diagnostic analysis of a wanton woman thus resolves into a truer understanding of a wanton womb.

It is important to note here that Riverius's analysis is not based simply on a belief that body affects mind, that behavioral or mental disturbances have organic causes. Galenic medicine did not distinguish in any essential way between psychic and somatic conditions and it was therefore entirely normative to treat by material means conditions such as womb fury or melancholy or the spleen that a later medicine would categorize as more purely psychological. The issue is rather that in describing this particular ailment, Riverius exploits the Galenic tendency to subjectify the parts to give prominence to the womb over any sense of a holistic person. The woman who madly seeks after copulation turns out to be a ravenous womb writ large.

This pattern of the womb's occlusion of the woman (the part taking precedence over the whole) typifies as well the contemporary understanding of "fits of the mother," also called "suffocation of the mother" or "hysteria," the protean condition anciently ascribed to a wandering womb but in the seventeenth century understood to arise either from more localized movements of the womb within the abdomen or from the noxious vapors emerging from retained seed.[26] The condition itself had numerous manifestations, from immobility and seeming cessation of respiration to convulsive fits, howling, and crying. Edward Jorden describes the symptoms as "monstrous and terrible to beholde, and of such a varietie as they can hardly be comprehended within any method or bounds."[27] With no precise description and yet encompassing so many different and contradictory ailments, the disease was as amorphous as it was debilitating. In its most extreme forms, hysteria makes manifest what these books on women's healthcare generally convey, though not quite as explicitly as here, that the workings of the womb overtake the possibility of a rationally and autonomously volitional female subject.

A central assumption underlying writing about the fits of the mother is that during such a fit the patient is at the mercy of her raging womb. The idea works physiologically because the womb was understood to have a "wondrous sympathy," as Crooke says, with all other parts of the body. The womb therefore affects and is affected by all that happens both in the body's principal parts, namely brain, heart, and liver, and in the animal, vital, and natural faculties with which those parts are affiliated. In fits of the mother, therefore, as Jorden explains, "all the faculties of the bodie doe suffer; not as one may do from another, but all directly from this one fountaine, in such sort as you shall often tymes perceyve in one and the same person diuerse accidents of contrarie natures to concurre at once" (*BD*, 1 v). The functioning of the entire organism can therefore be affected—from our ability to "vnderstand, judge, and remember things that are profitable or hurtfull vnto vs" (*BD*, 11 v) to our (involuntary) ability properly to digest and excrete food. Jorden wrote his brief discourse to argue for a womb-based etiology for the disease against lay opinion that its symptoms could be caused only by demonic possession. But in detailing the manifestations of the disease, Jorden portrays the raging agency of the womb rather than any specific sense of a separable female subject possessed of a problematic body part.

Having the typical capacity of certain body parts to perceive their own condition, the womb, Jorden explains, can "find . . . it selfe anoyed by some vnkind humor" and will therefore "communicate" the "offence" to "the rest of the body" (*BD*, 6 r). The result of such communication can encompass an inability to speak, to hear, to move, to feel, to see, to remember; the potential result, in other words, is total debilitation or erasure of a volitional person.[28]

The womb's rhetorical ascendancy, not as the paramount part of a woman's body but as a synecdoche for woman herself, is most explicit in the stories of women mistakenly taken for dead who were in fact only suffering from fits. Although they were not unique to him, Jorden tells of one such story

which Ambrose Paree reporteth of Vesalius a worthie Physition, and for anatomicall dissections much renowned, who being called to the opening of a Gentlewoman in Spaine, which was thought to be dead through the violence of one of these fits, began to open her, and at the second cut of the knife she cried out, and stirred her limbes, shewing manifest signe of life to remaine. (*BD*, 11 r)

When Crooke tells a similar story, he finds in it the somatic ground for the common truth of women's untrustworthiness:

In my time there went a woman begging about this Citie, who had a Coffin carried with her, and oftentimes she fell into those Hystericall fits, and would lye so long in them, nothing differing from a dead carkasse, till the wonted time of her reviving. Hence it may be came the Proverbe, *Thou shalt not believe a woman . . . no not when shee is dead,* till she be buried. (*M*, 225)

Woman's propensity to lie is here conflated with the body's "lying" about its vitality. These stories make explicit the both the womb's subsumption of the subject and, reciprocally, the ease with which the characteristics of woman's "nature" (women lie) are written onto the womb and its effects.

The treatments recommended for women suffering from these fits appropriately perpetuate this conflation. Here is Riverius's suggestion:

The sick party must be laid upon a bed in such a posture, that her Neck and Shoulders lie high and sloaping, but her Thighs and Privy parts lie low and shooting downwards, for so the Womb is more easily reduced.

Then must her lower parts be tied very hard, so as to cause pain; likewise they must be well rubbed and chafed; also Cupping-glasses are to be set upon her Hips; and a very large Cupping-glass set upon her Share is very profitable. But take heed that you do not apply a Cupping-glass upon the Patients Navil, which many ignorantly are wont to do, for by that means the Womb is drawn upwards again. (*PP*, 426)

Riverius assumes that fits of the mother routinely arise when the womb "is removed out of its proper place" and so "must be restored to the same again" (*PP*, 426). Yet the logic of the cure attends to the "sick party" more than to her womb. The problem with a womb "removed out of its proper place" is that it is not sufficiently "bridled," in Crooke's terms, yet what gets tied down here is not the womb, but the woman; the physician must tie her down very hard, so as to cause pain. The woman and the womb seem to be interchangeable; the proper response to a propensity to stray, in wombs as in women, is to enforce by artificial means the constraint that is not evident in the creature by nature. Riverius can recommend tying down the woman when it is the womb that needs to be bridled, because the woman and the womb are one.

Traditional and popular Galenic therapeutics for women's diseases thus replicate and perpetuate the same assumptions about female personhood that we saw elaborated in the much more philosophically-oriented biology of Crooke's *Microcosmographia*. Across genres and throughout a century, physiologically as well as therapeutically, woman was conceived of as an extrapolation of the womb rather than as a person possessed of a characteristic part. The anxieties and illogicalities attending the meanings and use of medical knowledge about women in the instructional manuals of the time mark the troubled status of the female, so much so, that the unified and agential subjectivity conveyed so clearly by the genre gets undercut, subsumed in the function and diseases of the womb.

In the years after 1651, Galenism increasingly fell under attack, both by the empirical discoveries of the new methods of observation and experimentation and by the growing popularity of chemical medicine and mechanical philosophy. Despite these challenges, however, the models of gendered subjectivity generated in early modern texts of Galenic medicine managed to survive; in fact, as the next two chapters will show, in writings regarding new research in embryology, they even managed to intensify.

# MODERN MODULATIONS

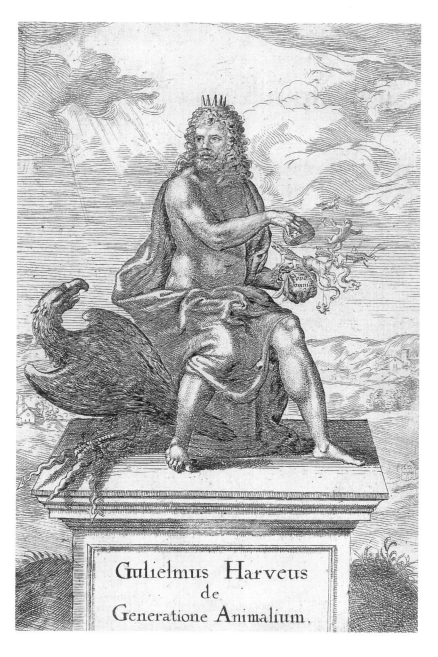

Plate 5. *Frontispiece of William Harvey's* De generatione animalium *(London, 1651),
depicting Zeus opening an egg, from which all life derives.  Reproduced by permission of
the Harvey Cushing/John Hay Whitney Medical Library of Yale University.*

## 4 / *Making Up for Losses:*

### *The Workings of Gender in Harvey's*
### De generatione animalium

**B**Y REPEATED DISSECTION OF HEN AND DEER IN the 1630s and 1640s, William Harvey determined, erroneously, as it turns out, that there is no mass, either of mixed semina or of male semen and female menstrual blood, to be found in the uterus after intercourse. Although *De generatione animalium* is famous for much else, it seems fairly clear that Harvey considered this experimental discovery momentous because it unambiguously demonstrated to him that all his predecessors, who had assumed the existence of some postcoital mass, had drawn "false, and rash assertions" about the origins of generation.[1] Harvey's empirical method was once again successful, as it had been in his discovery of the circulation of the blood, both in banishing what Harvey called the "clouds" from traditional knowledge and in establishing a sure foundation for new theories of animal physiology (*DG*, a5r).

Historians of science have evaluated the accuracy of the conclusions that Harvey drew from his observational discovery, particularly the roles he assigned to the male and female in procreation and the status he accorded to the egg produced.[2] But precisely because it deals explicitly with male and female procreative agency, Harvey's text may profitably be studied in terms of its more or less implicit constructions of gendered identity. Harvey's discovery of the absence of any postcoital mass in the uterus was indeed revolutionary, not merely because it contravened the biological teachings of Aristotle or Galen but also because it threatened to contravene the certain knowledge of male dominion, in both the family and the state, with which those theories had historically been aligned. Starting from an observationally produced "fact," Harvey suggested a theory of generation that simultaneously endorsed and enabled contemporary configurations both of gendered subjectivity and of the hierarchical relation between the sexes. Although his central physiological proposals did run counter to the prevailing theories of the time, his efforts to conceptualize and describe them reveal a deep cultural embeddedness, for Harvey's language works consistently on the one hand to preserve the pattern of gender relations assumed by earlier theories and on the other to inscribe onto the biological processes he studies a newly emerging (and distinctly modern) notion of man.

■ In turning to Harvey's *De generatione animalium*, our study now shifts from a focus on derivative texts, translations, and compilations, many written by now-forgotten figures who were important in their own day primarily for reformulating ancient traditions, to the learned discourse of a man universally famous in the history of medicine and commonly called the father of modern physiology. We shift now, therefore, not only to original, even revolutionary, research but also to original prose, to the work of a physician and natural philosopher seeking to articulate and evaluate a new understanding of a crucial and mysterious aspect of animal and human physiology. This shift to studied prose affords an opportunity to examine the interlacing of what to us may seem to be distinct semantic fields. For Harvey, who worked and wrote during a time of unprecedented political turmoil in his country, ideas of bodily organization are inseparable from ideas of political structure and, as we shall see, his understanding of the self emerges equally from both discursive domains.

The overlap between discourses of the body and of the body politic is not, of course, unique to Harvey. The analogous relation between body and state is at least as old as Plato and it was not uncommon, in Harvey's day as in ancient times, to describe one in terms of the other.[3] Thus it made sense for Dr. Walter Charleton to propose in a treatise on nutrition and digestion written in 1659 that "the most perfect Model or form of Government . . . is the Body of Man," and for James Harrington, a parliamentarian opposed to Harvey's ardent Royalism, nonetheless to cite Harvey's work on the circulation as the basis for his utopian vision of a republican state, an intellectual effort he referred to specifically as a "political anatomy."[4] Perhaps the best known instance of the explanatory force of bodily structure in justifying the structure of a state is the so-called Fable of the Belly, of ancient origin but popularized in Harvey's period by the character Menenius Agrippa in Shakespeare's *Coriolanus*, who argues for the entitlements of the aristocracy by recounting a fable in which rebellious bodily members come to recognize their dependence on the centralized governance of the belly.

Pervasive as it was in the texts of the time, the homology between body and state, as John Rogers has rightly pointed out, is not simply a literary device but a deeply entrenched pattern of conception and explanation. In both political and natural philosophy it was crucial to understand how the structure of the body/ body politic was organized, what caused it to change, and under what kind of authority it changed. The natural science of bodies and the study of the body politic were discursively interdependent because they were conceptually so: the same kinds of questions animated each field of inquiry and, often enough, writers cast their conclusions about one in terms appropriate to the other.[5]

The overlap between physiology and political structure in Harvey is perhaps most evident in his work on the circulation of the blood. Harvey dedicated the first edition of *De motu cordis* (1628) to King Charles, and in his dedication he asked his sovereign to "contemplate the Principle of Mans Body, and the Image of your Kingly Power."[6] Though surely a form of flattery, the analogy does have explanatory force, for Harvey explicitly conceives of the body's physiological organization as a monarchy, working under the beneficent dominion of the centralized authority of the heart. The heart, Harvey explains, circulates the blood throughout the body and is thus responsible for the body's sustenance; it is therefore rightly thought of as the "Prince" within all creatures, the "Sun of their Microcosm . . . from whence all vigor and strength does flow." Likewise, he explains, "the King is the foundation of his Kingdoms, the Sun of his microcosm, the *Heart* of his Common-Wealth, from whence all power and mercy proceeds."[7] Like the King in his Commonwealth, the heart in the body is the fount from which "all power in the animal is derived."[8]

As much as Harvey's model of the heart as the reigning organ responsible for distributing life-giving blood to the body aligns with ideas of hierarchical organization befitting a monarchy, his fundamental commitment to vitalism, which, as various scholars have noted, entails a more "republican" rhetoric, exists in tension with this conceptualization.[9] As Rogers explains, when Harvey published his second treatise on circulation in 1649, he emphasized the blood's self-motive, vital quality; circulation occurred not simply from the pumping force of the heart, but more emphatically from the self-moving agency of the blood. The heart, dethroned, as it were, from its position of central authority, now becomes "serviceable" to the needs of the self-circulating blood, which Harvey refers to as "the fountain of Life."[10] Even though Harvey himself was a Royalist, considered politically, vitalism has what Rogers calls a "radical tug," because it assumes the self-reliant, literal vitality of noncentralized aspects of an organism. Harvey's vitalism further promotes an idea of the organism as physiologically autonomous over and against its environment because the organism's system works by a self-enclosed and self-impelled circulation. Far removed from Galen's "passible" self fully enfolded in its environs, Harvey's understanding of the circulation and of the blood coheres with early modern notions of the self as an autonomous individual, what Rogers explicitly identifies as a protoliberal subject.[11]

Rogers does mention Harvey's *De generatione* in his study of the "vitalist moment" in seventeenth-century England, but only briefly, and only insofar as it bears on his understanding of *De motu cordis*, which constitutes his primary focus. But politics and physiology are also very much at issue in *De generatione* and it is there that Harvey treats, physically as well as conceptually, the formation of the individual organism and the origin of animal life. It is therefore to that text that we turn to study Harvey's particular interlacing of the rhetorics of body, polis, and self.

■ In considering the cultural inscriptions of *De generatione*, it is important to remember that Harvey arrived at his theory of generation in a highly politicized context. As personal physician to Charles I, Harvey conducted some of his most definitive experiments on the king's lands and at the king's behest; although *De generatione* was probably written during the second half of the 1640s, when the king was already held captive by parliamentary forces, it was based on work performed for the most part in the 1630s.[12] For years, Harvey was connected to an increasingly embattled court whose king was engaged in an ultimately unsuccessful struggle to maintain his patriarchal rights over his subjects. While the prefatory matter of the 1651 text argues Harvey's distance from the turmoil of the time, the contention that scientific study was a much needed refuge from the "anxious cares" of the day suggests Harvey's keen awareness of the politicized context in which he worked. The clearest evidence of the cultural embeddedness of Harvey's work is that his discovery of the postcoital absence of semen in the uterus neatly replicates the threat to political patriarchy that surrounded him. According to classic patriarchal arguments, the king rules his kingdom as a father rules his children; political and paternal rights were understood to be analogous or even synonymous.[13] As King James argued in *The Trew Law of Free Monarchies*, "By the Law of Nature the King becomes a naturall Father to all his Leiges at his Coronation: And as the Father by his fatherly duty is bound to care for the nourishing, education, and virtuous government of his children; even so is the King Bound to care for all his subjects."[14]

Harvey's determination that the semen has no material contact with the egg surely threatens the nature of paternity, since without physical continuity between father and fetus the role of the father in generating the fetus becomes ambiguous. But it also threatens the nature of patriarchy as a form of civil government, since classical patriarchy, the theory that political right is paternal right, depended, at least implicitly, on the transmission of that right through paternal procreation. Although patriarchal arguments took many forms in the seventeenth century, a common ground of evidence was found in the biblical account of God giving Adam dominion over his wife and children. As Richard Field argued in 1606, "When there were no more in the World but the first man whom God made out of the earth, the first woman that was made of man, and the children which GOD had given them, who could be fitter to rule and direct, than the man for whose sake the woman was created, and out of whose loynes the children came?"[15]

Ignoring the first Creation story, in which male and female are created simultaneously (Genesis 1:26–27) and erasing entirely the female capacity for birth, Field founds Adam's rule on his status as the sole material source of procreation: Eve derives from his body and the children from his loins. Implicit in Field's argument is the biological assumption that the father exclusively creates the child: from *his* body, from *his* loins. Although clearly an inversion of the obvious, that children come from a women's loins, Field's position, which was common to patriarchal arguments, was actually supported by both Aristotelian and Galenic physiology, which granted the father the greater share of procreative agency.[16]

The partriarchalists' use of Eve's derivation from Adam's body to support claims of paternal rule offers perhaps an exaggerated example of how both biblical stories and biological theories can get enlisted in political argument. When patriarchal writers spoke of rulers in general and not specifically of Adam's rule, however, the connection between generative and political sovereignty could not be explicitly made, since kings could not be said literally to father their subjects. Nonetheless, the connection between paternity and patriarchy continued to function in their claims, if only figuratively. Sir Robert Filmer, for example, founded the right of governance in God's original granting of paternal power to Adam, and he demonstrated that this power descended only through Adam (not through Eve) because as "the Scripture teacheth us . . . all men came by succession, and generation from one man."[17] But because Filmer recognized that political right was not always transferred by lineal descent—kings could be usurped, for example, or governments consolidated—he did not actually rest his argument for patriarchy on the physiology of paternity.[18] That the two were nonetheless linked in his theory is evident from his telling response to Hobbes's contention that in the state of nature children owe their original obligation to their mother. This could not be, argued Filmer, because we know "that God at the creation gave the sovereignty to the man over the woman, as being the nobler and principal agent in generation."[19] Because Adam, as *man*, is the "principal agent in generation," he achieves solitary rule over both wife and children, and it is on the basis of that physiological model that we are to understand the paternal rule of kings.[20]

Patriarchal theory in the seventeenth century had grounds of support other than the biology of paternity, but if an analogy between the two was at least implicitly embedded in claims for fatherly rule, then Harvey's discovery, which threatened the traditional understanding of paternity, also threatened the understanding of patriarchy that derived from the father's procreative superiority.[21] Harvey's responses to the two conceptual dangers posed by his experimental work are, however, somewhat different from each other. While he mitigates the threat to paternity by playing out a fantasy of exaggerated male dominion, he counters the threat to patriarchy by transmuting it to a dominion based in a broadly masculine, as opposed to a specifically paternal, right.[22] This emerges in Harvey's depiction of the embryo as an autonomous, freeborn male, unbounded by any constraints to either father or mother. In stressing the embryo's masculine autonomy, an autonomy that, as we shall see, characterizes Harvey's endeavors as an empirical researcher as well, Harvey's theory bears certain similarities to the famous myth of origins envisioned by his good friend Thomas Hobbes, who published his own work of anatomy and masculine birth, *Leviathan*, in 1651, the same year that Harvey published *De generatione*. For both theorists, masculine right reemerges as traditional patriarchy gives way, and the masculine, freeborn individual becomes the basis of the modern state.

■ *De generatione* is set up as a series of exercises, some detailing Harvey's findings from various dissections and observations and some presenting the speculative conclusions he drew from them. Although Harvey never sets forth a formal or systematic theory of embryogenesis—in fact, *De generatione* is deemed valuable in the history of medicine less for its positive formulations than for its rejection of prior theories—he does provide ideas toward a theory, speculations and observations that, though they never quite cohere, represent his thinking about what he called nature's "Closet-secrets" (*DG*, a6v).[23] Working from his determination that there is no semen to be found in the uterus after intercourse, Harvey reasoned that fertilization must occur without the semen having material contact with the egg. For Harvey, it is important to note, the "egg" was not what we refer to as the ovum but, rather, the complete origin of the embryo, produced solely by the female; if the female was fertilized through intercourse, the egg would develop and grow on its own, either within the female's body (in viviparous animals) or outside it (in oviparous ones).[24] When Harvey asserted that all living things comes from eggs (as the frontispiece of *De generatione* depicts, see plate 5 on page 100), he was not propounding a universal female contribution from an ovary but was rather suggesting that oviparous, rather than viviparous animals should be understood as the paradigm case for understanding generation. (Harvey thought that the ovary in viviparous animals did not participate in the process of generation at all.)[25]

Although *De generatione* follows Aristotle's teaching in much else, Harvey's discovery of the lack of semen in the uterus compelled him to differ from Aristotle, as well as from Galen, with respect to the components of conception.[26] For Aristotle, the semen acted directly on the female menstrual clot and, though contributing nothing material to the future embryo, actually was responsible for forming it and for determining its *telos*; the female, by contrast, supplied the matter on which the semen worked to craft the offspring. Aristotle's analogy for this interaction makes the point: the semen works on the menstrual material as a carpenter does on a tree, carving out its creation from some prior matter.[27] In Aristotle's theory, the female's role as material cause allows her to be rightly considered a parent of the offspring, but it is the male contribution that provides the motion of the offspring and directs its formation, and, so, it is the male that is considered the primary progenitor.

The Galenic theory, which vied with Aristotle's for roughly 1,500 years, differed from Aristotle's in attributing procreative seed to the female. But Galen concurred with Aristotle in deeming the female's role to be vastly inferior to that of the male. Because of the hierarchic homology between male and female reproductive parts, the seed produced from females' testes, was, as we have seen in previous chapters, necessarily inferior in quality and importance to the seed produced by the more perfect organs of males. As Thomas Raynalde wrote in his edition of *The Byrth of Mankynde*, "the seede and sparme" of woman is not as "stronge, ferme, and mighty in operation as the seede of man"; it is, rather, "weke, fluy, cold, and moyst, and of no grete fyrmitie" (*R.BM*, 14v–15r).

As numerous recent scholars have shown, both Aristotle's and Galen's embryological theories align contemporary biological knowledge with prevailing assumptions about gender relations.[28] Harvey's discovery that these theories misconstrued the makeup of the material body of the fetus threatened to topple their corresponding assumptions about gender because it undermined their biological support: if there is no postcoital mass in the uterus, the semen cannot be considered to contribute directly to the fetus. Further, the female must be seen to produce *on her own* the egg out of which the fetus develops. Harvey certainly considered the possibility of female preeminence in generation. He reasoned that since a hen can produce unfruitful eggs without the cock, and since these eggs clearly have some vital principle that propels them from the ovary through the uterus, "all power of Production, or the Soul [*anima*] doth not proceed from the Male" (*DG*, 160–61). Harvey even refers to the female as an efficient, and not merely material, cause of generation, and he looks to Aristotle to support his assertion that the female may even be considered the primary agent in generation:

> [I]t seemes probable, that the Female is a stronger party in Generation, then the Male: For *in the Universe likewise, the Earth is held to be, as it were, the Female and the Mother: But the Heavens and the Sun, and the other Bodies of that kind, Philosophers call by the name of Father and Genitor* ([Aristotle] *De generatione animalium* 1.l.c.2). Now the Earth also produceth many things of its own accord, without any Seed: And amongst Animals, some Females do procreate of themselves without a Male; (thus the Henne generates a Subventaneous Egge) but the Male never begetteth any thing without a Female. (*DG*, 161–62)

As the male role in procreation fades into indeterminacy, the female's role emerges, at least potentially, as predominant.

It is important to understand that Harvey *needed* to assert female agency to explain how an egg can be produced without the semen's material contribution to its development. But the potential of that agency's really assuming preeminence over the male was troublesome; if the female herself were considered to control the giving of life to the egg, the traditional association of male with spirit and female with matter might be reversed. John Rogers has argued that just such a transformation is in fact inevitable, given Harvey's commitment to vitalism. Because in vitalism matter itself is spiritualized, vitalism "work[s] inevitably to elevate the discursive category of femaleness" and, he argues further, "to necessitate a feminism."[29] It is my contention to the contrary that it is precisely because of the threat of this "elevation"—a threat implicated as much by Harvey's observational discovery as by his physiological theory—that his rhetoric works so hard to contain it. Harvey, of course, never portrays his discovery as potentially threatening in this way; his repeated assertions of his empirical findings bespeak his pride and confidence in the efficacy of diligent observation in the unveiling of truth. But although it is possible to read his occasional statements of female agency in procreation as indications of his willingness to alter the established gender hierarchy, the sense that the prospect was in some fundamental way actually inconceivable to him is registered in the elaborate edifice of explanation that Harvey constructs to counteract both its biological and social implications.

Forced by his discovery into believing that the semen had to act at a distance in order to have any role in generation, Harvey confessed himself unable to determine definitively how fertilization occurs. But it was a problem that fascinated him, one, he said, which was "indeed a dark, obscure business," with much that he thought "worthy our wonder" (*DG*, 539). Harvey even included in *De generatione* an appendix devoted exclusively to the problem of conception, so that it would not appear that he "onely goe[s] about to subvert other mens opinions, but also to disclose our owne" (ibid.). Unable to establish any empirical evidence for the process of fertilization, Harvey attempted to figure its workings through analogies. He presents these analogies without apparent order, each useful in part but none adequate to the task of fully conceptualizing the process he strives to describe. Taken together, though, they do cohere as something of a logical sequence, one that works to foreclose the possibility of female control in generation and to entrench instead male preeminence by progressively reassociating the female with matter and the male with the pervasive power of spirit.

The first in the series, though not the first to appear in the text, is the suggestion that the semen works like a magnet:

> And because it is certaine, that the Geniture of the Male doth not so much as reach to the cavity of the Uterus, much less abide there for any time; . . . the Woman or Female doth seem after the spermatical contact (in coition) to be . . . rendered prolifical, by no sensible corporeal Agent, as the Iron touched by the Loadstone, is presently indowed with the virtue of the Loadstone, and doth draw other iron-bodies unto it. Namely, having once received that virtue, which we have spoken of, it doth exercise the plastick generative power, and procreateth its own like, no otherwise then plants doe, which we see are impowered with the force of both sexes. (*DG*, 539–40)

Of all the analogies Harvey uses, this one most aligns the male with materiality and the female with procreative agency. The semen here is considered the vehicle of an incorporeal "plastick generative power," but the process necessitates a material "touch" to transfer that power to the female. Once fecundated, though, the female is said to be able to produce a being after *her* "own like"; through a derivative power, she is given the capacity to re-create *her* own form. It is fairly clear, however, that Harvey was not satisfied with this understanding of fertilization, since he mentions it only a few times.

Another analogy, Harvey's most frequent and the one that apparently made most sense to him as a physician, is that the semen acts like a disease, propagating by contagion.[30] Conception should be understood to occur, Harvey suggests, in the same manner in which "Contagious, Epidemical, and Pestilential Diseases . . . do foment and disperse their infection through the air, and propagate distempers like to themselves in other bodies, and by a secret course, as it were, by a solemne generation tacitly multiply" (*DG*, 206).

The contagion idea is useful to Harvey's purposes partly because it helps to explain the multiple births typical of many animals, and also because it demonstrates the irresistible, exclusive, and multiplicative vigor of the semen. Scattering his seed, the male is still a material cause here. But, unlike in the magnet analogy, it is the male who here re-creates *his* image. In fact, every time Harvey mentions the contagion idea, he suggests that the generative ability belongs exclusively to the male; he says, to cite another instance, that animals are "begotten as it were *per contagium aliquod*, by a kind of contagion. In like manner as Physitians observe, that contagious diseases . . . do propagate their infection, and beget themselves in bodies yet sound and untouch, merely by an extrinsical contact; nay sometimes onely by the breath . . . and that at a distance, through an inanimate medium, and that medium no way sensibly altered" (*DG*, 254). In marked counterpoint to the male, who, by analogy, "beget[s] [him]sel[f]," the female is figured simply as the place of propagation, as the passive recipient of the male's powerful touch.

Whatever its explanatory advantages, however, the analogy to contagion did not really accommodate all the particularities of Harvey's understanding of generation. In Harvey's theory, the female is not a wholly passive recipient; by whatever means, she does actively produce the egg. Perhaps recognizing the disjunction, Harvey devotes most of his appendix on conception to explaining a third analogy, in which uterine conception is understood in terms of mental conception. He starts from the observation that the inner surface of the uterus, when ready to conceive, "answer[s] in lubricity and softness to the internal ventricles of the Braine" (*DG*, 542). Based on this physical resemblance, and on the double meaning of *conception*, Harvey reasons there must exist a functional resemblance as well. Because, he says,

> the substance of the Uterus, now ready for Conception, doth so nearly resemble the Constitution of the Braine: why may we not imagine, that both their functions are also alike; and that something like, if not the selfe same thing that the phantasme, or appetite is to the brain, is excited in the Uterus: from which the generation or procreation of the Egge doth succeed? for both their functions are equally called conceptions, and both are Immaterial; though they be the principles of all the actions of the body. . . . And as Appetite doth spring from the conception of the braine, and that conception from the outward appetible or desirable objects, So also from the Male (as being the more perfect Animal) as from the most natural appetible object, the natural conception doth arise in the Uterus, as the Animal conception in the Brain. And from this Appetite or Conception is commeth to pass, that the female doth produce an offspring like the male Genitor. (*DG*, 542–43)

Though starting from a consideration of uterine conception, this analogy works to magnify the male, asserting his association with the incorporeal. As "the most natural appetible object," the male procreates nonmaterially, imparting to the female an "idea" or "form" of himself through intercourse. Only in response to that incorporeal influence can the female conceive the egg. Furthermore, although the female is said to "produce an offspring," the offspring is said to be "like the male Genitor," not like the mother, as it was in the analogy to magnetism.[31]

The last of the analogies completes Harvey's complex balancing act between a female who *must* be said to produce and a male who nonetheless *can* be said to be the primary creator. In this analogy, Harvey takes to their logical extreme the complementary concepts of the male as both "idea" and "the most natural appetible object": here, the semen functions as the original creator, God:

> What it is, that is *hoc Traducis*, this Derived essence, which cannot be perceived to be either remaining, or touching, nor any sensible contained thing; and yet doth operate with a vast discretion and providence, beyond all the bounds of Art: & which doth render the Egg prolifical, even when it selfe is fled and vanished, not because it now doth, or hath touched before; not fructifying only the perfect, and absolved eggs, but even the imperfect and intended only, when they are yet but whelks and pushes: nay

the Henne her self, before she have yet produced any whelks at all, and that so nimbly, as if the Almighty himself should say, Let there be a production, and strait there is one. . . . In the generation of things is seen the most excellent, the eternal and almighty God. (*DG*, 205–7)

In this analogy, the semen resembles God in the first moments of the universe, creating by fiat. By mimicking the divine "Let there be light," Harvey's "Let there be a production" gives to the semen all life-power of creation; the female produces germs of eggs, but they become fruitful, they are endowed with life, only through the agency of the semen. Harvey even suggests the female's awareness of the semen's divinity, since the hen, he observes, after intercourse, "(as one ravished with delight) shakes her feathers for joy, and as if she grew proud from the Boone she received, composeth and rectifieth all her extravagant Plumes: like one that adored the deity for the grand benediction of multiplying issues" (*DG*, 175–76). Here, finally, is the realigned balance of matter and spirit. The female produces material eggs, but the male alone gives them the spark of life, for which the female viscerally gives thanks. Although confessing himself "at a stand" (*DG*, 548), Harvey considers the function of semen that must work from afar and he sees, finally, God.

Taken together, Harvey's analogies reveal his difficulties with the prospect of denying to the semen the formative function possible with the old notion of persistent material contact between male and female contributions to generation. Harvey's conclusion (which he shared with his teacher, Fabricius) that no material contact was involved in embryogenesis is surely polyvalent: it could mean that the semen controlled the process from a distance, but it could also mean that the semen was merely a mechanical trigger, and that life, form, and substance were all imparted to the egg by the female. Harvey's analogies strive to foreclose the possibility of the latter by progressively giving to the male all the control in the generation of life.

Harvey in fact sees male predominance in generation not only in the possible explanations for the mechanics of fertilization but even in the act of intercourse itself. *De generatione* is filled with sex stories, from traditional lore about female animals that died for lack of regular intercourse to graphically detailed accounts of heterosexual and even homosexual mating practices. Like fertilization, sexual practice was a topic that fascinated Harvey—he even planned a future volume called *The Loves, Lusts and Sexual Acts of Animals*—and, as with his consideration of fertilization, he found in it ample evidence of male dominion. What is particularly interesting in his accounts of male sexual prowess among animals, however, is his consistent and unabashed anthropomorphizing; whereas in his writings about fertilization, the connection to human beings is implicit (based on the idea that oviparous generation is the model for viviparous generation), in his discussions of animal sexual behavior, Harvey routinely speaks of a cock's "wives" or the desire of doe to protect their "chastity." The result, at least rhetorically, is an implied analogy between the sex life of animals and that of humans, so that the practices that appear as normative among one cannot be thought of as wholly foreign to the other.

Although *De generatione* includes some evidence of female "lustiness," Harvey attends more closely to male sexual aggression, and he repeatedly describes scenes of animal rape. For example, we hear of

> a Cock-Pheasant, penned up in an aviary, [which] boils with such scorching lust, that unless he have severall hennes with him, (six at the lest) he will extremely afflict them with repeated Coitions, and rather retard their fertility, then promote it. I once saw a Pheasant-henne, so spent and worn out by the cocke who was shut up with her (whom she could no wayes escape; neither by flight, nor concealment) that her back was grown bald by his frequent accents, until at last, in miserable torture, she expired for grief. (*DG*, 32–33)

The females, for their part, are "compelled to submit" to the males' advances, and they are accounted to incite the males' desire whether or not they are actually inclined toward sex: "[S]ometimes the coyness and morosity of the Hen doth not a little conduce to rouse and heighten the males sleepy heat, and languishing appetite, to quicken and encourage his performance" (*DG*, 202–3). Harvey presumably includes this observation to demonstrate that females may, in certain respects, be considered a "first cause" of generation, but the implication is that the females get sex whether or not they want it. Similarly, Harvey tells the story of a gander "who, wanting a mate, sojourned with the hennes, where his lust was so unbounded, that for some hours together he pursued a young pullet withersoever she fled, arresting her with his bill, till at length he triumphed upon her weariness, and subdued her to a Rape" (*DG*, 33). The most straightforward understanding here is that rape is both natural and normative, performed as evidence of power, and not only of the male over the female but between males themselves. Thus Harvey tells us that a common "dung-hill cock having gotten the mastery in [a] duel, doth sate his desires not only upon the concubines of his foe, but upon the conquered himselfe" (ibid.). In this instance, the purpose of sex is not to procreate (which is how Harvey generally portrays it elsewhere) but rather to demonstrate dominion. That Harvey anthropomorphizes here as elsewhere (the cock's "concubines") suggests that he thought of these animal sexual patterns as not wholly alien to human relations; sex is a power play, and females, whatever their desires, are mostly the objects of rape.

Harvey's treatment of the male role in generation, both in the act of intercourse and in the process of fertilization, seems at pains to establish the pervasiveness of male prowess; the male is constructed as a sexual conqueror, dominating his partners and endlessly regenerating himself in them. But Harvey also needed explicitly to treat the female role in generation and here he met again with a threat to normative gender relations, since the female had to be responsible for producing the egg without direct contribution from the semen. If *De generatione* alleviates that threat on the male side through analogies that realign the male with the giving of life and through descriptions of male sexual behavior that unambiguously demonstrate male dominance, it deals with the threat on the female side by nearly erasing her importance, particularly in relation to the being she produces.

Harvey explicitly curtails the possibility of female predominance by taking back his assertions of her procreative agency. For example, just one page after asserting that "the Female is actually a stronger party in Generation then the Male" (*DG*, 161), he corrects himself, as it were, to assert that she is "as eminent" as he (*DG*, 162). But, of course, the female cannot really be *as* eminent as the male, as Harvey makes clear in his discussion of female physiology. Even as he rejects the Galenic position of females as inferior versions of males, Harvey manages to maintain the physiological insufficiency of the female in embryogenesis (especially in viviparous animals). In exercise 34, Harvey argues against the Galenic position that females, like males, emit spermatic liquid at orgasm and that it is from the mingling of these two semina that conception occurs. His evidence is threefold: first, he says, not all prolific female animals, and certainly not all childbearing women, experience such emission; second, the liquid is emitted primarily externally, that is, at the orifice of the vulva and never within the uterus, so, it could not be mingled with the male emission, which enters the uterus more directly (*DG*, 172–76). It would seem that either of these arguments would suffice to cripple the Galenic position. But Harvey's third argument, the one he apparently feels is the most forceful, derives from his already certain knowledge that female physiology cannot attain to the perfection of the male and, so, cannot be said to produce what the male body can: "But for my part I wonder much, how they fansie, that so elaborate, concocted, and quickening a Semen, can arise from so imperfect and obscure parts [as the ovaries]" (*DG*, 175). The Galenic position is ultimately wrong, Harvey believes, because it is illogical to think that the female can match the male. And elsewhere, Harvey praises the arrangement of nature to produce perfection by supplying males to compensate for inherent female "failings":

> For in animals (whose Sexes are distinct) it is so contrived, that because the female cannot alone generate, nourish, & protect the foetus, the male is joined as yoke-fellow in the task (as the Superior, and more eminent progenitor) to supply her failings; and so to correct the infirmity of the Subventaneous eggs, and inspire them with fertility. (*DG*, 259)

There is no question here of symmetry, no sense that nature requires both and equally a male and a female to perpetuate a kind; rather, the male exists as the "Superior . . . progenitor" to correct a female failing.

In depicting the female as physiologically inferior to the male, Harvey's work corresponds precisely to the gender assumptions of his predecessors (though for different reasons). But Harvey also shows himself able to break from the teachings of the past while nonetheless maintaining its gender hierarchy; this is clearest in his treatment of the egg. Here the implicit project of *De generatione* to aggrandize the father and reduce the mother coalesces, for Harvey makes the offspring the exclusive image of the father, constructed on the near denial of the mother.

Harvey stands enraptured before the egg. It is, he says, "a period . . . of eternity," standing at the midpoint between those who are, those who were, and those who are about to be (*DG*, 137). Like God, it encapsulates the beginning, the middle, and the end of things: it marks the beginning of life, the mean between male and female, and the end of procreation (*DG*, 137–38). In determining the origin of the chick in the egg, Harvey is therefore delving into what he considers nature's greatest mystery; he says it is no easier to "discover the secret recesses, and dark principles of Generation, then the method of the fabrick and composure of the whole world" (*DG*, 76). It is important to note this consistent tone of radical amazement in Harvey's search for ultimate origins because it indicates the value he places on what he finds, namely the egg's abiding and near complete independence from its mother. He asserts this independence in all phases of the egg's existence: in its initial appearance in the uterus, in its ability to grow and develop into a fetus, and in its eventual birth. In each of these phases, the egg functions on its own as a vital, autonomous entity.

This independence is first established in viviparous animals in the egg's emergence in the uterus. In all things relating to generation other than the function of the ovaries, Harvey insists on the analogy between oviparous and viviparous animals. But whereas he was able to chart with some specificity both the periodic changes in the hen's ovaries and the day-to-day changes in the incubating egg, Harvey could not do the same for the viviparous ovary or embryo. He could not see any change in the viviparous ovary before or after intercourse, and he could not see anything resembling a yolk. The "eggs," which Harvey describes as masses resembling pudding appended to the uterus, seem to spring up, as it were, of their own volition six to seven weeks after intercourse (*DG*, 419ff.); from their first appearance, the eggs of viviparous animals seem to have no essential connection to the mother. The mother's role as efficient cause in generation reads as if reduced to nothing; the embryo just suddenly appears, as if on its own.

Once visible, whether as a yolk in hens or as a conception in doe, the egg proceeds to develop by its own power. Harvey agrees with Fabricius that the function of the uterus is to produce and grow eggs, but he stresses that growth occurs not by means of the uterus but "proceedeth . . . from an innate natural principle of its own" (*DG*, 45). In other words, the embryo, vital from its first beginnings, is responsible for its own development. To make the point, Harvey emphasizes that even while it is within the fowl and connected with the ovaries, the hen's egg may not, "be said to be a Part of its mother, nor to take life and vegetation from her soul, but from its own proper power, and intrinsecal principle" (*DG*, 143). The vital principle that controls the growth of the egg is proper, intrinsic, to the egg itself.

This idea of the egg's self-regulation and innate vital principle is one of Harvey's most remarkable breaks with Aristotle and is the central point of his entire understanding of the embryo. For Aristotle, the semen formed a fetus out of menstrual blood, endowing it with a vital principle that would direct its growth. But for Harvey, nothing external to the egg is responsible for its vitality; the *anima* is essentially the egg's own. In explaining the process of epigenesis, the doctrine that growth and development happen simultaneously, Harvey uses the analogy of a potter, whose work takes form and increases at the same time. Unlike the artificer who "cuts and divides the matter which is provided to his hands, and so by paring away the superfluous parts, doth leave an Image remaining behinde, as the Statuary doth," the potter "formes the like Image of Clay, by adding more stuff, or augmenting, and so fashioning it, so that at one and the same time, he provides, prepares, fits, and applies his materials" (*DG*, 222). Unlike Aristotle's analogy between generation and an artificer's work, Harvey's analogy is inexact because, embryologically, there is in his theory no distinction between the potter and his creation (thus, the potter cannot be the semen, which never touches the egg). The egg must therefore be understood to make itself. Though he retains the Aristotelian vocabulary and way of thinking about what constitutes an explanation, Harvey undoes the Aristotelian distinction between formal and material causes in the embryo; for him, the embryo both en-forms *and* en-matters itself.

This sense of the egg as a self-made entity is bolstered by the metaphors and similes that Harvey routinely uses to describe its autonomy. Not surprisingly, Harvey understands the egg's self-determination in particularly gendered terms. The egg, he says, "(even while it is contained in the Ovary) doth not live by the Soul of the Henne; but is a freeborn, Independent Issue from its very first original" (*DG*, 145). Again, in arguing that the egg is "neither the Workmanship of the Uterus, nor controuled or governed by it," Harvey thinks in terms of sons freed from the control of their parents; the egg, he says, "tumbles and roules in its Cavity free, and disjoined (like a Son who hath obtained his Freedom) and growes up to perfection" (*DG*, 150). "[L]ike a Son come to age, and at his own dispose, [eggs] are regulated and enliven'd by their own proper soul" (*DG*, 151). Even in Harvey's other analogy for the autonomy of the egg, which compares eggs to the seeds of plants, seeds are said to be perfected "in the womb of the earth by an internal vegetative principle" (that is, they are not controlled by the tree) (*DG*, 150); "being dis-united from the Plants," the seeds "are no more accounted parts of them" (*DG*, 151).

Since Harvey conceives of the egg's autonomy as a release from some prior bondage, like a son freed from parental control, and since the egg's only previous connection is to the mother that produces it, that freedom is gained by separation from her. Here again, the radical autonomy of the egg can best be seen in contrast to Aristotle, for whom the identity or essence of the embryo is carried by the male, who constitutes the offspring's formal cause. In establishing the egg's identity, Harvey breaks with the Aristotelian pattern by making the embryo self-determining. Because the embryo is self-motive, its identity is generated in and by itself; the embryo becomes the very paradigm of the self-subjectifying man. Because of the implied threat of female control of fetal growth and development that Harvey's initial discovery makes possible, this emphasis on self-regulation and self-determination assumes special importance in Harvey's scheme. Though surely an effect of Harvey's vitalist assumptions, the emphasis on an autonomy metaphorized as a son freed from the mother reads at least in part as a safeguard response to the conceptual threat of maternal control.

Just as the egg becomes for Harvey a full and vital creature from its first appearance, the mother, in turn, becomes a fetal incubator, even while gestating her offspring. This is equally true of viviparous and oviparous females, since Harvey considered the uterus an internal nest, the place where the egg is "cherished, ripened, and hatched into a foetus" (*DG*, 5). Even the act of birth is a wholly passive process for the mother, since the fetus, both fowl and human, releases itself from its place of growth. In describing the oviparous birth process, Harvey notes that shell fragments are propelled outside the egg; this demonstrates, against Fabricius, that the chick essentially hatches itself from its shell. Working again on the idea that oviparous processes are the model cases for viviparous ones, Harvey then makes the analogy to human beings: the human fetus "himself sets open the Gates of the Womb with his head turned downward, and unlocks their inclosure by his own force, and so struggleth himself into the world by conquest" (*DG*, 490). Though Harvey recognizes the occasional efforts of the womb, the "greater part" of birth is the work of the fetus, not of the mother. Battling its way out of its confinement, the fetus works alone and without aid.

To press the point, Harvey tells two stories, of which he says he has personal knowledge. In the first he recounts the case of a woman in his village whose child was born the morning after the woman died. Though the woman was dead the night before, Harvey explains, "an Infant was there found between her Leggs, which had by his own force wrought his release" (*DG*, 492). The second story is rather more grotesque but more forthright in its implications:

I also knew a Woman, who had all the interiour part of the neck of her Womb excoriated and torne, by a difficult and painful delivery: so that her time of Lying in being over, though she proved with Child again afterward, yet not onely the sides of the Orifice of the Neck of the Womb and the Nymphae did close together, but all the whole Cavity thereof, even to the inner Orifice of the Matrix, whereby there was no entrance even for a small probe, nor yet any egress to her usual fluxes. Hereupon the time of her delivery being now arrived, the poor soul was lamentably tortured, and laying aside all expectation of being delivered, she resigned up her keys to her Husband, and settling her affairs in order, she took leave of all her friends. When behold, beyond expectation, by the strong contest of a very lusty Infant, the whole tract was forced open, and she was miraculously delivered; the lusty Child proving the author of his own, and his Parents life. (*DG*, 492–93)

The effect of Harvey's story emerges clearly in contrast to Jonas's comment in his edition of *The Byrth of Mankynde* some hundred years earlier. Whereas Jonas fashions the mother, in her patient Christ-like suffering, as the deliverer of mankind, Harvey reverses the roles; here it is the son who is the deliverer, the purveyor of miracles, a hero who brings life even to those on the cusp of death.[32]

What emerges, then, from Harvey's treatment of embryology is that the mother's role in generation, while initially active, is only fleetingly so; she generates the egg but is unconnected to it. Yet this fleeting agency is crucial to the definition of what become the two *male* roles in procreation. In producing the egg but then being separate from it, the mother at once allows the father's role to be conceived of as godlike and allows the egg to be seen as wholly independent and self-determining and thereby as decidedly masculine, as a "son" at "his own dispose" (*DG*, 151). Acting for only a restricted period between the injection of divine semen and the arising of the self-reliant embryo, the mother becomes that against which males define themselves and in relation to which males grow; for the father she is a place in which to reproduce himself and for the embryo a place to find comfort and nutrition. In other words, perhaps not surprisingly, the mother in Harvey's theory serves biologically the roles that she was beginning to serve socially in the emerging bourgeois household. When Harvey therefore looks to the "secrets" of generation, he sees what surrounds him: self-sufficing and independent males and the females whose function it is to promote them.

Harvey's depiction of the embryo's radical autonomy and masculine identity formation in the socialized terms of a son who comes of age takes on special significance in the context of the times in which he wrote, when debates about subjection to paternal authority were carried out on the battlefield. In the early 1640s, Harvey's friend Thomas Hobbes challenged the natural origin of paternal political right, in part by turning to biology. In Hobbes's state of nature, dominion follows from the physical fact that females give birth. Since, he says, it cannot be known who the father of a child is except by the testimony of the mother, and since the mother has it in her power either to nourish the child or to expose it to the elements, the child "is therefore obliged to obey her, rather than any other; and by consequence the Dominion over it is hers."[33] Though this perhaps sounds promising as the basis of a protofeminist politics, feminist critics have shown that Hobbes's interest in mother-right inheres less in establishing the dominion of females, or even an enduring equality between men and women, in the state of nature than in countering patriarchal arguments: originary mother-right is a way to deny the natural rights of the father and thus of any civil ruler.[34] But mother-right is a fleeting moment in Hobbes's thought; useful as a critique of the argument that paternal right is natural, it quickly gives way to a collection of radically autonomous individuals. Although Hobbes is never explicit about how such individuals become free—at one point in *De Cive* he simply asks his readers to consider individuals as if they were sprung up like mushrooms[35]—the state clearly arises from a social contract among free men, not those subject to parents.

It is a logical corollary to Hobbes's theory that if the individuals who contract into the state are wholly autonomous, self-driven, and self-regulating, they must achieve their identity and their independence in their separation from their original obligation to the mother. In tracing such a pattern of psychological development in Hobbes's individual, Christine Di Stefano sees the contours of modern masculine identity, an identity forged in negative relation to the mother. "The strict differentiation of self from others, identity conceived in exclusionary terms, and perceived threats to an ego thus conceived . . . all recapitulate issues encountered and constructed in the process of securing a masculine identity vis-à-vis the female maternal presence."[36]

While I do not wish to argue influence or even agreement on matters either political or physiological, I do want to note a confluence between the construction of the Hobbesian man and that of Harvey's egg. Just as mother-right is necessary but fleeting in Hobbes's theory, and just as the Hobbesian individual achieves freedom when mother-right is superseded, Harvey's egg achieves its independence in its separation from the mother who is said initially to produce it; like Hobbes's individual in the state of nature, Harvey's egg is self-determining and wholly autonomous.

Of course, for Hobbes the postulated past of radical freedom is necessary to justify the legitimate rights of a de facto state—the myth of prior freedom justifies subjection to Leviathan's sword—whereas, for Harvey, the autonomy of the individual seems genuine and enduring. But for both, writing in the mid-seventeenth century in the midst of the greatest social upheaval their country had ever known, the originary human being—in the state of nature for Hobbes and in the mother's womb for Harvey—is autonomous, self-ruled, and distinctly masculine.

The similarity between these two theorists inheres not just in their construction of an insular identity, however; it obtains on a more directly political and public level as well. In studying the contemporary debates between the classical patriarchalists, who identified political with paternal right, and the emerging social contract theorists, who considered political right to be derived from the consent of freeborn individuals, Carole Pateman has argued that patriarchy itself did not so much die out in the seventeenth century as get transformed. Recognizing that patriarchy proclaims man's dominion as both father *and* husband, Pateman suggests that the contract theorists rejected paternal right but "simultaneously transformed conjugal, masculine patriarchal right."[37] Pateman argues, for example, that Hobbes is a "patriarchalist who rejects paternal right": whereas mother-right provides a counter to paternal right, it does not provide a counter to masculine right, since even in the state of nature, Hobbes speaks of families in which the husband unambiguously rules.[38] She shows the crucial transitional role of originary mother-right, which denies paternal right as natural, yet coexists with masculine or conjugal right. Hobbes's civil state is therefore postpaternal but not postpatriarchal.

In light of Pateman's analysis of Hobbes, Harvey's innovative treatment of the egg as an autonomous individual reads as a physiological version of the same process that Hobbes recorded in his political theory—the transition enacted during the seventeenth century from a patriarchy based on paternity to one founded on masculine right made manifest in the mastery, and self-mastery, of the male individual. If the traditional physiologies held the father to be the prime creator and thereby supported the understanding of the father as the origin of political power, Harvey's discovery, in jeopardizing the father's role in generation, jeopardized its political implications as well. But rather than reassert the old patriarchy, as he did paternity, Harvey substitutes for it the independence of the egg, the new, self-made and self-enclosed man, and thereby replicates the political process of his time: from monarchy to commonwealth, from paternal control to independent male sovereignty.

■ I have been arguing that, given the dangers to sexual and political ideologies posed by his initial discovery, Harvey variously re-creates masculine supremacy in the outlines of his embryological theory and in the rhetoric of his text. It is perhaps inevitable that Harvey encodes the same pattern of self-determining masculinity in his depiction of his own efforts as a scientist; the Harvey that emerges in *De generatione* is autonomous, heroic, and even, at times, godlike. Although Harvey follows both Aristotle and Fabricius in many points, and in fact strives wherever possible to align his observations with their opinions, he routinely takes pride in demonstrating his independence from them, in showing them wrong. In fact, Harvey opens *De generatione* with just such a declaration of independence:

> Since many have requested, and some have importuned mee; it will not, I hope, be unwelcome, (candid Reader) if what I have observed concerning the Generation of Animals, out of Anatomical dissections (for I have found the whole matter to be much different, from that which is delivered, either by Philosophers or Physitians) I expose in these Exercitations, in favour, and for the use of the Lovers of Truth. (*DG*, a4 v)

There follows a brief statement of the Aristotelian and Galenic positions on embryogenesis, and then Harvey continues:

> But that these are false, and rash assertions, will soon appear; and will like clouds instantly vanish, (when the light of Anatomical dissection breaks forth). (*DG*, a5 r)

Harvey here presents himself as the torchbearer, breaking free from the shackles of traditional knowledge, driving away the old bogeys of his predecessors. Just as the egg is characterized as a son freed from maternal bonds, so too is Harvey a son freed from the bonds of his teachers.

Further on in his introduction, Harvey takes on the role of hero-adventurer, a role commonly assumed by early modern scientists, in which the experimenter explores and seeks to control some uncharted and typically feminized territory.[39] Arguing for the difficult method of direct observation over the more popular but indolent habit of reading books, Harvey says that discoveries have been made only by those who, "following Natures conduct with their own eyes, have at length through a perplexed but yet a most faithful tract, attained to the highest pitch of Truth. And in such an undertaking it is pleasant, not to be tyred onely, but even to faint away; where the Irkesomness of Discovering is abundantly recompensed by the discovery it selfe" (*DG*, a6r).

The rhetorical suggestion of science as an arduous but ultimately pleasing pursuit takes on a slightly sexualized significance in the context of Harvey's particular subject matter, not only because the territory he will claim is the female body itself (and not merely a more abstracted feminized nature) but also because his role in achieving dominion over it is characterized by the same aggression and violence that he will elsewhere describe as typical in male animal sexuality. Describing the external genitalia of the common fowl, Harvey explains that the three orifices of the pudenda are "vailed by the labra of the privity, and the parts called Nymphae; so that, without dissection, or at lest some forcible retraction of that covering, neither the passage of the Excrements out of the guts, nor of the Urine out of the Ureters, nor of the Egg out of the Uterus, can appear in a Hen (*DG*, 17). This is Harvey's only mention in *De generatione* of the "forcible" method of dissection, and it is telling that it comes in the context of a unique description of a sexual encounter in which the fowl reveals herself in the same position as the dissected fowl is revealed before Harvey, that is, with pudenda exposed to sight:

> [I]n coition, the Hen unvaileth her lap, and accommodateth it for the Cock that treadeth her. . . . I have seen an Ostrich-Hen (when her Keeper gently stroked her back, with designe to inflame her) groveling on the ground, lift aside that vaile, and expose and stretch out her lappe; which the Cock perceiving, being instantly cupid-struct, proceeded to tread her; and having one leg on the ground, and the other on her back, with an exceeding large Yard (of the dimensions almost of a Neats-tongue) pursued his attempt: great was the noise and clamours on both sides, and their necks often extended and retracted, and many other expressions of content. (*DG*, 17)

With the use of a knife and a "some[what] forcible" exposure of parts, Harvey displays before himself the pudenda of the fowl in the same way that she readies herself before the cock for sex. In this description—and this is rare in *De generatione*—the male's approach is seen specifically to be gentle, and the female herself presents her parts for his approach. There is then an odd kind of parallel between Harvey and his scientific subject on the one hand and the cock and his sexual mate on the other. It is as if the female's voluntary self-exposure compensates for the force of Harvey's heroic methods, the "exceeding large Yard," an instrument of apparent pleasure, displacing the less pleasurable exposure to a knife.[40] That violence, however, also declares Harvey's dominion not only over the subject itself, the body of the female fowl, but over his subject matter more generally, for the forcible use of the knife is, as Harvey explains in his introduction, the "perplexed [and] most faithful" way of achieving truth.

Finally, Harvey finds in his work a moment of godlike power. In the course of his research, Harvey has noticed that the *punctum saliens*, the little beating bit of blood that is the first sign of a chick embryo, stops its motion when removed from incubating warmth but returns again to life when some manner of heat is reapplied:

> [E]xpose an egge too long to the colder aire, and the Punctum saliens beats slower, and hath a languishing motion; but lay your finger warm upon it, or cherish it kindely any other way, and it presently gaineth strength and vigour. And after this Punctum hath declined by degrees, and being full of blood hath ceased from all motion, exhibiting no specimen of life at all, and was given up for lost, and dead, upon laying of my finger warm upon it, for the space of only twenty pulses, the poor heart hath awaked, and recovered again, and as it were rescued from the grave, proceeds to its former harmony afresh . . . as if it were in our dispose to condemne the little Soule to the Shades, or reprieve it to life, at pleasure. (*DG*, 95)

Such power to bring a "poor heart" back from the Shades—literally to control life and death—is surely superhuman and is a most distinctive mark of Harvey's self-inscription as the idealized, and even godlike, masculine subject.

Yet for all Harvey's heroic posturing, he cannot, as he freely admits, penetrate to the mysterious center of generation. In this, too, he mimics the semen, unable to enter the inner sanctum of the womb, where the secrets of life abide. This final similarity, grounded as it is in apparent inadequacy, suggests something about the nature of the idealized images of masculinity that pervade Harvey's text. The godlike semen, the conquering cock, the autonomous egg, the heroic researcher—they are all constructed in response to perceived or threatened failures, of paternity and patriarchy as well as of the empirical method of science, which finally cannot tell Harvey how embryogenesis happens. The images of masculine triumph therefore appear somehow compromised, generated not from their own vital power but, like the egg itself, from a perceived absence. Seen in this way, the workings of gender in Harvey's *De generatione* can never make up for losses; they can only expose them to view.

## 5 / Embryonic Individuals:

## Mechanism, Embryology, and Modern Man

SOME TIME IN 1672, THEODORE KERCKRING, A Dutch physician and microscopist, autopsied the body of a woman who had died three or four days after her period. On opening her uterus, Kerckring found "a little round mass the bigness of a black cherry."[1] Having determined from the widower that he had had relations with his wife within a few days of her death, Kerckring asked permission to "take the cherry home" so that he might investigate it further. When he dissected his specimen, Kerckring discovered something amazing: "nature," he said, "had wrought with so much activity in so small a time that one might already see the first lineaments of a child, since we observed in [the cherry] the head as distinct from the Body, and in the head we took notice of some traces of its principle organs."[2]

Kerckring's discovery was reported in *Philosophical Transactions of the Royal Society*, as a part of its English-language review of his recent work on fetal osteology. Although Kerckring explicitly claims to have observed only "the first lineaments of a child" in his "black cherry," in the rest of the report on his research, he is quoted as emphasizing the early morphological completeness of embryos in general; by one month, he says, a conception "has the whole human shape, and the Bones thereof firm enough in many places to support the parts."[3] Yet, despite his exclusive concentration on the physiological question of fetal development as opposed to the more philosophical or theological issue of ensoulment, Kerckring is nonetheless at pains to refer to this incipient organism as a "child," even as an "infant."

Kerckring's sense of the embryo as a complete child, as opposed to merely a complete shape, is especially evident in his illustrations of early fetal development.

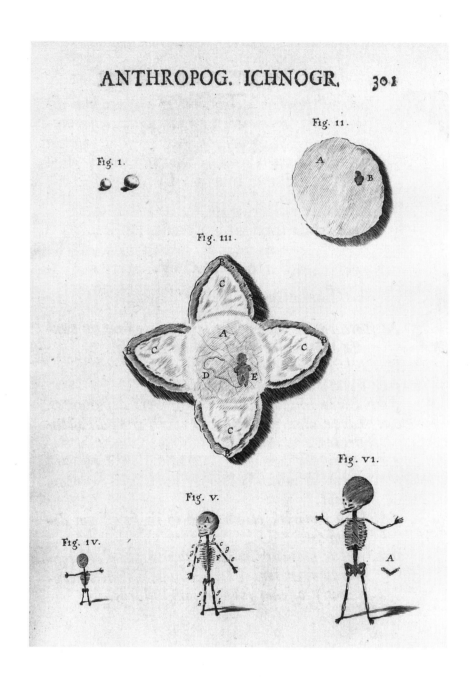

*Plate 6. From Theodore Kerckring's* Opera omnia anatomica *(1717),*
*the plate depicts early fetal development.*

Figure ii of plate 6, which shows what Kerckring found in his three-day-old cherry, offers a miniature emerging upwards from a plane; though no internal organs are visible, one can discern the "child's" facial features fairly distinctly. Figure iii, which represents an "egg" opened two weeks after conception, portrays a figure without features but with clearly delineated limbs. Figures iv through vi illustrate the skeletons of what Kerckring explicitly calls "infants" three, four, and six weeks after conception. All of them stand not only upright but in rather expressive postures. Other than growing in size, the only difference between the six-week-old and the three-week-old is that the older "child" seems ready for social interaction; given his posture and facial bearing, one might suppose him to be in the midst of a conversation with some absent partner. Taken together, the figures are seemingly imbued not only with structural completeness but with some sense of personhood. The implication of embryonic personhood is all the more remarkable because Kerckring relied on a theory of generation that suggested that procreation was essentially a mechanical process. The vitalism that had, literally, animated Harvey's understanding of the body and its processes had fallen increasingly out of favor during the second half of the seventeenth century. For Kerckring, as for many others at the time, the coming-to-be of a new organism could be explained according to the laws of matter and motion; he thus refers to the one-month-old "child" as a "self-sustaining engine."[4]

Neither of the ideas manifest in the journal report—the personhood of the embryo and the embryo as a machine—was unique to Kerckring; both were, rather, part of the larger landscape of theoretical and empirical embryology of the later seventeenth century, during the course of which theorists increasingly looked to mechanism for an explanatory framework through which to understand the process of the development and growth of organisms. At the same time, however, the theories they proposed asserted the emergence of distinctive and coherent identity at ever earlier points in the process of generation—thus Kerckring's willingness to designate a three-day-old embryo a child. The result, during the last half of the century, is an inverse relation between the extent to which a theory is indebted to mechanism and the length of time before the entity created can be said to exist as identifiably itself: the more mechanistic the theory, the earlier the attribution of identity. Though generally dismissive of (or oblivious to) Harvey's vitalism, these theories seem to want to maintain vitalism's implications for identity—a self-determining, self-motive organism that is identifiably itself from the appearance of the first speck of beating blood. Vitalism may be dismissed in the mechanistic theories this chapter studies, but the person remains.

The embryology debates of the seventeenth and eighteenth centuries have been subjected to contextual analysis in numerous works on the history of generation, but most of them chart the embeddedness of the theories in the explicit philosophical or religious concerns of the time.[5] Given the formulation in which an embryo can be deemed both an infant and a machine, however, it seems apparent that theories of embryogeny also engage questions about the contours of human identity, of what defines it as such, whence it derives, and what its specific characteristics are. It is my argument here that the competing theories of embryogenesis and the conflicting formulations of the embryo itself in the decades after Harvey take part in the conceptual struggles accompanying the emergence of the early modern individual.

■ The gradual mechanization of embryology in the late seventeenth century was part of a more general interest in mechanical physiology that was then gaining the attention of medical researchers in both England and on the Continent. In 1637, Descartes had declared the human body "a mere mechanical contrivance"; by 1663, Boyle was able to claim that the "human body itself seems to be but an engine, wherein almost, if not more than almost, all the actions common to men with other animals are performed mechanically."[6] In turn, the mechanization of the body took part in the increasing use of mechanical metaphors to understand all manner of human and natural processes. Thus in the analogous realm of the body politic, man was understood as being susceptible to mechanical, mathematical analysis. From Hobbes's building of the artificial man of *Leviathan* to William Petty's reduction of the body politic to a quantifiable mass, man was understood in both his physiological and social functions as a mechanical being. One way to understand the emergence of embryos as little engines, therefore, is to see it in confluence not only with mechanical physiology but with social visions such as those of Hobbes and Petty. Just as subjects within a state operate invariably according to specific "natural" laws (enabling the possibility of a predictive political *science*), so the human embryo functions as a machine, an engine that labors in its own growth in regular and predictable ways but is not, and logically cannot be, self-regulating or individualized.

In their commitment to mechanical explanation, Kerckring's mechanical embryo, Boyle's body engine, and Petty's body politic all share in a cognitive heritage that is frequently framed as dualist. Descartes's rationalism, his rending of the body from the domain of the thinking soul, is perhaps the clearest example of such dualism, but Baconian empiricism, too, which characterized so much of the practice of the new philosophy in late-seventeenth-century England, proposed an enforceable boundary between the unencumbered mind of the scientist and the material world he studied. In his early vision of a new science, Bacon had even ensured the objectivity of experiment by claiming that "the whole business [would] be done as if by machinery": science would proceed strictly by applying the experimental method to neutral cases so that the process of discovery would be protected by the boundary that the experiment would putatively enforce between bodily distortion and cognitive clarity.[7]

The researcher of the late seventeenth century, then, both physiological and social, turned a disembodied gaze on an inanimate world. Though surely dualist from one perspective, it is possible also to see in the relationship between intellect and matter a vision of the early modern subject itself: the unencumbered mind of the scientist gestures toward the autonomous, self-determining subject of liberal individualism and social contract theory; the regularized machine of the body he studies points to the undifferentiated anonymity of political economy and early demographics. These two poles—of subjectivity, agency, and autonomy, on the one hand, and anonymity, mechanism, and determinism, on the other—together characterize the tensions in emerging notions of selfhood.

The same uneasy interconnection that holds between the rational subject and the inanimate object is evident, too, in the very term *mechanism*, which came to stand synecdochally for so much of the new philosophy in the seventeenth century. Though frequently counterposed to the human, the *mechanical* in its seventeenth-century usage actually presupposed it: a "mechanick" was one who engaged in manual labor, such as an artisan or craftsman, and *machine* frequently had the meaning of tool or device, that is, something that needed to be worked with the hands.[8] But however much the mechanical was already associated with the human, the relation between the two was also vexed because, although in some sense human, the mechanical could not be *fully* human. In other words, the mechanical was necessarily *merely* mechanical, since it referred to manual as opposed to rational labor. Thus Henry Peacham warned in *The Compleat Gentleman* that "Painting in Oyle . . . is . . . of more esteeme than working in water colours; but then it is more mechanique, and will rob you of over much time from your more excellent studies."[9] The mechanical man, the mechanical body, thus, always threatened to be just that and no more.[10]

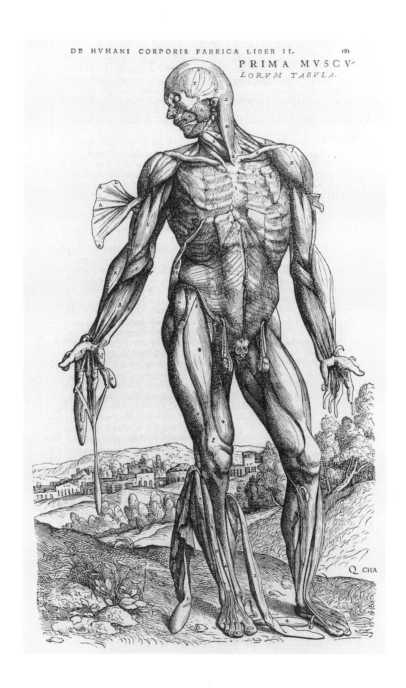

PRIMA MVSCV-
*LORVM TABVLA.*

Q CHA

*Plate 7. From Vesalius's* De humani corporis fabrica *(Basel, 1543),*
*the plate depicts a "muscle man" in an animated posture of display.*

This inextricable but troubled relation between anonymity and subjectivity, between the mechanical and the human, is neatly displayed in sixteenth- and seventeenth-century anatomy texts, many of which include representations of the human cadaver in postures of "living anatomy" or self-dissection (see plate 7). Jonathan Sawday, in his exploration of what he calls the Renaissance "culture of dissection," suggests that such images indicate a remarkable "acquiescence . . . a willing participation on the part of the anatomized subject."[11] Sawday reads these life-in-death images as an effort to mitigate the anxiety aroused by the necessary violence of dissection and by the anatomist's own implication in "the grim business" of acquiring bodies to dissect, since these might be thought to compromise the truth status of the anatomy's results. "So," he argues, "instead of an anatomy being performed *on* the body of a recently executed criminal, the illustrations show us a corpse conspiring with its own demonstrations, in order to confess the truth of the study which has been embarked upon"[12] Sawday understands the typical placement of these cadavers in rural or domestic frames as a sign both of the imputed "naturalness of dissection" and of the cadavers' participation in a lesson about human destiny: "*et in arcadia ego*—'Even in Arcadia there am I, Death.'"[13] But beyond signifying something about the moral and epistemological status of the endeavor, the illustrations suggest something about the body itself as well; the paradoxical liveliness of the cadavers, some of which appear in postures of ecstasy or seem to be caught in mid-stride, suggests an insistence on the body as an animated form, as if in an attempt to counter the reduction of the body to the mere physical structure presupposed by anatomy. If the culture of dissection sought to know the human body by its material form, and thus called into play the sense of the body as passive matter, it also needed to mitigate that conclusion by displaying the body, even in death, as vital and volitional— that is, as a *subject*.

A similar sense of troubled identity pervades the embryological theories of the seventeenth century. Just as the anatomical illustrations testify to a tension between undifferentiated and subjectified visions of man, so the very embryological theories that foster engine-like embryos. with one important exception, strive in their rhetorical formulations to individuate them, to grant them coherent, recognizable identities, and, in one theory, even to subjectify them. Thus Kerckring's black cherry is figured as an engine but with unsettling urgency is claimed to be a child. The urgency of the reiterated claim suggests something of a compensatory response; despite professions of wonder over the intricate complexity of the human engine, the threat of a truly mechanical man haunts the theories that describe him. The theories' rhetoric, as it selectively and differently allots identity status to the various agents involved in generation—father, mother, and fetus—demonstrates the resistance to the reduction of the origins of the human self to mechanical artifice.

■   The first thing to say about the personhood of Kerckring's embryo is that it is new. Whatever the innovation of referring to a bit of the body as an engine, Kerckring's characterization of a month-old conception as an infant or a child goes against both ancient and even contemporary knowledge about fetal status in the earliest stages of its existence. That there was a long tradition resisting the personhood of the fetus before quickening is evidenced in the history of the legal treatment of abortion. Legal subjectification of the fetus is a relatively recent phenomenon. Prior to 1803, which saw the enactment of Lord Ellenborough's Act, common law restricted abortion only after quickening, or perceived fetal movement, which, according to traditional manuals on pregnancy and childbirth, would occur some time between the third and fifth months of gestation.[14] Medieval church documents frequently distinguished between early and late "abortions," referring to early states of the fetus as "unformed" or "in a liquid state," and to early abortions, therefore, as not deserving of the same punishment as an abortion performed later in the pregnancy. Some sacramentaria referred to antifertility measures as "homicide," but they still did not treat the "sin" in the same category as premeditated murder. John Riddle, who has studied the history of contraception and abortion in the West, cites an Irish penitential from c. 800 that assigns increasing levels of penance for pregnancy terminations performed during the three stages of fetal development—establishment in the womb; formation of the flesh; and ensoulment.[15] Positions such as these derive ultimately from an ancient distinction between the time before and the time after the fetus is formed, which allowed Aristotle, for one, to suggest, in describing an ideal city on the verge of overpopulation, that abortions be induced "before sense and life have begun in the embryo."[16] Evidently, Aristotle assumed that the embryo could exist in some sense without actually being alive.

This distinction is borne out in seventeenth-century common law, too. Edward Coke, in *The Third Part of the Institutes of the Laws of England* (1644) asserted

If a woman be quick with child, and by a Potion or otherwise killeth it in her wombe; or if a man beat her, whereby the child dieth in her body, and she is delivered of a dead childe, this is a great misprison and no murder.

As Angus McLaren notes in his study of the "reproductive rituals" in early modern England, Coke is actually relaxing here earlier common law declarations that *did* consider a precipitated miscarriage to be murder.[17] But in all cases through the eighteenth century, the qualifying criterion for punishment, whether for murder or a "great misprison," or for something less grievous, is that the woman be "quick with child."[18]

Early modern herbals and medical manuals similarly seem to assume a divide between the statuses of a conception before and after quickening. Many manuals openly discuss, and explicitly condemn, "abortion," but by and large the term is used to indicate only pregnancy terminations that follow quickening. And, despite the abhorrence of abortion, there are frequent discussions of "bringing down the flowers" or "provoking the terms." A 1544 herbal discusses savin and hellebore to "provoke the menses"; Sir Kenelm Digby encouraged sulphur of antimony to "bring down a woman's course."[19] Whether these remedies were intended exclusively for amenorrhea or whether they were quietly understood to be useful (and sanctioned) abortifacients in the early stages of pregnancy is perhaps debatable, but that they were recommended so routinely suggests a willingness to think it legitimate to restore regular periods to a woman whose periods had stopped without thinking of that act as the "killing" of a "child."

McLaren suggests that this distinction between the generally legitimate remedy of "provoking the terms" and the damnable practice of abortion has precisely to do with the meaning of quickening. Roughly analogous to Aristotelian "animation" and theological "ensoulment," quickening was the point at which "potential now became actual life."[20] He cites Jacques Guillemeau's assertion in his 1612 midwifery manual that a miscarriage before forty days is not an abortion but rather a "shift or a slipping away," and John Maubray's similar belief, over one hundred years later, that the fetus is formed around the fiftieth day but not animated until some time between the seventieth and the hundredth.[21] Whatever it was that existed at the beginning of fetal development, it was not, apparently, to be called a "child" or an "infant."

Aside from the question of quickening, another reason that midwifery manuals so routinely denied subject status to the embryo is that it was considered impossible to determine with any certainty that a woman was even pregnant. Books did list signs of conception but none was thought to be conclusive. A man might be told to consider whether he felt a sucking sensation on his yard, or a woman might feel a "quivering or shaking" at conception.[22] But a distended belly, as William Sermon warned in *The Ladies Companion*, could easily indicate "superfluous vapors and wind" and so should not be understood to necessarily signify a woman's being with child; Jane Sharp admitted that many of the rules were simply "too general" to be certainly proved in all women.[23] Part of the problem here was that many of the signs of conception, such as dimness of the eyes, pallor of the complexion, and a pervasive weakness of the body, suggested disease as much as pregnancy.[24] Even stoppage of the menses signified ambivalently: because the blood that would normally be shed through the menses would be used to feed the fetus, suppression of the menses could indicate a "true" conception; but it could also indicate an unhealthy stoppage caused by a "false" conception, such as an abnormal uterine growth, "a lump of flesh gathered together," commonly called a "mole."[25]

Even uroscopy proved ambivalent. Though there were numerous tests for conception based on the inspection of a woman's urine, writers did not agree on what within the specimen carried meaning or on the meaning of any one finding. William Sermon said that white streaks in the boiled urine of a woman indicated pregnancy; others said it showed the presence of a dead child.[26] Sharp suggested that if you kept a woman's urine for three days and then strained it through a linen cloth, you would know that she was with child if you found live worms in the cloth.[27] The variety of opinions, often offered within a single text, suggests that until the end of gestation, at the birth of a live infant, there was simply no certain way to determine whether what a woman harbored within her was a child or, rather, as one often-reprinted volume put it, "a foul mass of flesh that comes to no perfection."[28]

In such a conceptual context, the maternal body was understood to be opaque; given to ambiguous changes, it was ultimately uninterpretable. A woman's own expression of her somatic experience and not the physiological fact of a missed period was, therefore, the best register of her condition; as we saw in chapter 3, it was her perception of quickening that most reliably signified pregnancy. Though this, too, could sometimes be deceptive (since moles, occasionally, were known to move), still the best, most reliable register of whether or not a woman was pregnant before the actual birth was the woman's own sense that there was something "quick" within her.[29] That is, the woman alone was considered the subject of pregnancy. In an age before the emergence of obstetrics and its attendant technologies of fetoscopy, the fetus, especially in its early stages, was simply unavailable for elevation to personhood.

Yet even in these medical texts that spotlight the ambiguous experience of the possibly pregnant woman, one can notice suggestions of a contrasting discourse.

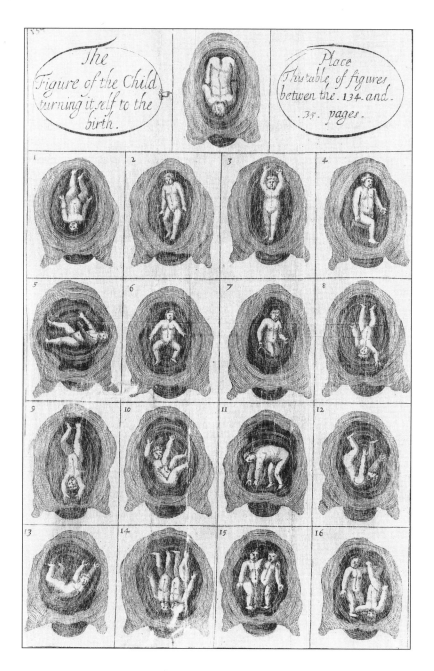

*Plate 8. From William Sermon's* The Ladies Companion, or, The English Midwife *(London, 1671), the plate depicts positions of the fetus in the womb. Reproduced by permission of the British Library.*

Many of the manuals written for midwives include illustrations of the various positions a fetus might take in the womb. Though putatively intended to help midwives understand the possible types of fetal presentation at birth, the illustrations also bespeak an understanding of the fetus and its relation to the body that bears it. Nearly all the images present the fetus as fully formed, floating in an isolated, dark space (plate 8). Perhaps in the context of the medical manuals, one can assume that that space is a uterus, but the illustrations themselves give no sense that the fetuses abide in a woman's body; they seem rather to be floating in oddly-shaped caves.[30] These stylized fetuses were conventional images of gynecological manuals, appearing in texts even hundreds of years before those that became popular in the later seventeenth century.[31] Occasionally, as in Jacob Rueff's *De Conceptu et Generatione Hominis* (London: E. Griffin 1637 [1554]) or James Wolveridge's *Speculum matricis hybernicum* (1670) (plate 9), the figures were presented with umbilical cords or were housed in containers that bore some semblance of an anatomical appendage, the ovaries, for example, but even then they appeared to be fully dissociated from the *materiality* of the woman's body; though some images suggested her *existence*, they almost uniformly denied her *presence*.

By schematically abstracting the fetus from its physical context within the woman's body, the illustrations allow the reader to see it—visually, but also conceptually—as an autonomous entity. In doing so, they allow a conceptual connection between the reader and the fetus that substitutes for the physiological connection between the fetus and the woman who carries it. In effect, these illustrations subjectify the fetus as an individual by silencing the woman, precisely inverting the maternal/fetal relation that the manuals otherwise present in discourse.

Analyzing these and other similar illustrations in her book on visual and verbal inscriptions of the fetus in early modern science, Karen Newman has noted the remarkable endurance of "the visual codes for representing obstetrical knowledge" from the middle ages through the seventeenth century, codes that promote fetal autonomy at the expense of the mother's intrinsic and active connection to her child.[32] But although the visual depiction of the personhood of the fetus *at term* is a centuries-old device, the seventeenth century offers for the first time in its embryology theories the personhood of the *embryo* and even, in one theory, of the generative germ.[33] For all their endurance, therefore, the images of fetal persons common to medical manuals resonate with a special significance in the seventeenth century because they intensify the implications of the new embryology, in both its theory and its practice.

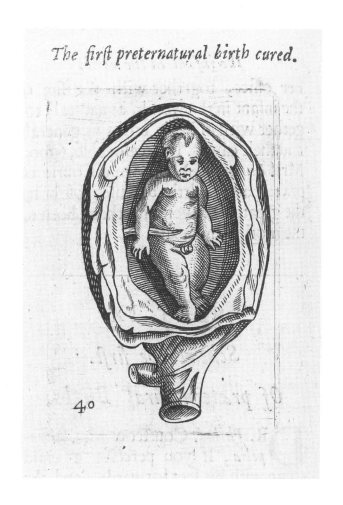

*Plate 9. From James Wolveridge,* Speculum matricis hybernicum; *or, the Irish Midwives* Handmaid *(London, 1670), the plate depicts a fetus positioned in the womb. Reproduced by permission of the Fales Library and Special Collections, New York University.*

One way to understand the emergence of embryonic subjects in the seventeenth century is to consider the practice of early modern embryology itself. Although people had been dissecting hens' eggs for the purposes of studying embryonic development for literally thousands of years, it was not until the late sixteenth century that embryology became systematic, and not until the second half of the seventeenth century that researchers such as Harvey and Malpighi charted embryonic development on a daily and even an hourly basis.[34] Furthermore, though much embryological research continued to be performed on hens' eggs, because they were cheap, plentiful, and thus easily available, increasingly in the seventeenth century, researchers were dissecting (and vivisecting) does, dogs, and rabbits to determine the nature of embryogenesis in quadrupeds. This latter research demonstrates most starkly the implications of dissection for maternal/fetal relations: one sacrifices the living maternal body to study the incipient fetal one.

Just as in the illustrations of the medical manuals, then, the empirical practice of embryology absents the mother from the arena of investigation, substituting for her the "living" presence of the unborn. Embryology thereby affords the researcher seemingly unmediated contact with his now "independent" object of study. And just as the illustrations of the medical manuals link the fetus conceptually with the reader rather than representing its physiological link with the woman who is carrying it, so in embryology, the visual contact between the scientist and the embryo established by the dissection of the maternal body (or its egg) lays the material groundwork for the conceptual subjectification of the fetus, only now, at its earliest stages, as an embryo.

If the practice of observational embryology therefore had something to do with the new rhetorical construction of the embryo in the seventeenth century, so too did the theoretical formulations that both guided and resulted from that empirical research. Because there was at the time no clear consensus on the meaning of what we would consider to be technical, classificatory terms, it might be best to begin with a sketch of the theories themselves. There were essentially four theories that arose roughly in sequence during the second half of the seventeenth century, each variously indebted to a waning vitalism and a growing commitment to mechanism.[35] The first, proposed in England in mechanistic form by Kenelm Digby and in vitalist form by William Harvey, was epigenesis, which posited the sequential production and development of embryonic parts from an originally homogenous substance. Metamorphosis, which Harvey had postulated for lower life forms like insects but which was adopted (and adapted) for higher organisms by Nathaniel Highmore and by later theorists such as Kerckring, asserted the simultaneous emergence of either all or the most important embryonic parts some time after conception. Preformation, the third theory, was similar to metamorphosis in that it asserted the original heterogeneity of the conception, but asserted that all the parts of the future organism were formed in the body of either one of its parents before conception; it thus pushed back the point at which the future organism could be (theoretically) identified in either the ovum or the animalcule. Preformation was perhaps the most widespread of the theories among academic circles at the end of the century, supported in its ovist form by George Garden and Reinier de Graaf, who first identified the existence of ovarian follicles in quadrupeds, and in its animalculist form by Anton von Leeuwenhoeck, who first announced the discovery of what we call sperm. The last of the four theories is now called pre-existence, which was most popular in the eighteenth century but had been suggested in the seventeenth. Pre-existence took the process even a step further back, asserting the existence of all parts of the future organism in miniature in either the egg or the sperm since the moment of the creation of the universe.[36]

For all their differences of physiological detail, the four theories shared an investment in questions of the etiology of human identity. No matter what the object of dissection, the question of human generation and human identity status was nearly always implicit in the embryological research of the time. Partly, this was a result of Harvey's work, which had argued that oviparous generation should be understood as the model for all generation; since, as Harvey famously claimed, all organisms come from eggs, one could study hens' eggs and learn something about human generation. As we saw in chapter 4, the famous statement on the frontispiece of *De generatione animalium*, *ex omnia ovo* was not an assertion of the existence of mammalian ova (in fact, Harvey thought the "testicles" in female quadrupeds were functionless) but rather a summation of Harvey's belief that the egg is the common original of all animals and therefore that all generation could be understood on the model of animals that hatch from eggs. Then, as now, such extrapolations across kinds were both quite common and considered scientifically valid.[37] In terms of generation theory, the effect was that even though much of the research was performed on hens' eggs and on quadrupeds, it was possible to construe its results as a template for human generation, if in somewhat less perfect form.

If analogical reasoning made possible certain hypothetical conclusions about human generation, however, it also worked to trouble the question of the human subject precisely because it necessarily blurred the line between the objects compared. This is particularly apparent in the work of Kenelm Digby, who, in 1644, offered a theory of mechanical epigenesis, that is, a theory that proposed the sequential production and development of embryonic parts by entirely mechanical means. His attempt to construct a mechanical theory of generation demonstrates the problems raised by analogical argument for the status of human identity, and, more broadly, by the application of mechanism itself to human generation.

A thinker much influenced by Cartesian dualism, Digby sought to explain the generation of animal bodies in purely mechanical terms, without recourse either to an innate vital spirit to direct the process or to the explicit intervention of God. What he came up with is a theory based on an analogy to the process of nutrition: just as, over time, ingested food changes by degrees into different substances that eventually merge into flesh and bone, so, Digby argues, "why should not the same juice, with the same progresse of heate and moysture . . . be converted at the first into flesh and bone though none be formerly there to joyne it self unto?"[38] Digby postulated that superfluous nutritive juices are reserved "in a fitt place" in the testicles of both males and females where they eventually coalesce into homogeneous substances. These substances, when joined together in coitus and when acted upon by various external forces such as heat and moisture, change over time and by degrees into a living creature. Digby therefore concludes that "all generation is made of a fitting, but remote, homogeneall compounded substance: upon which, outward Agents working in the due course of nature, do change it into an other substance, quite different from the first . . . [so that] by successive mutations . . . that substance [is] produced, which we consider in the periode of all these mutations" (*TT*, 218).

Although Digby recognizes that to believe that new creatures come from the body's excess food may be to stretch the limits of reason, he assures his readers that the proposition is quite credible if one thinks not of the two extremes of beginning (nutritive juice) and end (living organism), but rather of the step-by-step process of sequential change over time. He argues, in fact, that the transformation is actually inevitable, and he offers the example of plant development as an illustration: "Take a bean," he says,

> or any other seed and put it in the earth, and let water fall upon it; can it then choose but that the bean must swell? The bean swelling, can it choose but break the skin? The skin broken, can it choose . . . but push out more matter, and do that action

which we may call germinating? Can these germs choose but pierce the earth
in small strings, as they are able to make their way? (*TT*, 217)

Astonishingly, without elaboration, Digby then asserts the same process in sentient creatures, though presumably it would be performed "in a more perfect
manner, they being perfecter substances" (*TT*, 218).

In making so effortless an analogy between beans and sensible creatures, Digby
silently glosses over the important question of how sentience is generated, of
what *distinguishes* the generation of creatures from the generation of plants,
despite their similarities. The analogy becomes particularly sticky when the language Digby uses to describe the *necessity* of the bean's development is applied
to sensible creatures. The theory, as is clear from Digby's rhetoric, is thoroughly
deterministic, his emphasis throughout is on the force of necessity; the reader
is repeatedly asked if the bean "can choose but" that something be the case, suggesting and stressing the inevitability of the process. Since, in concert with his
mechanical assumptions, Digby wants to deny "a specific worker within" or a
"cunning artificer" who directs the development of an original homogenous mass
into a complex organism, the deterministic language is appropriate. But when
he makes the analogy to human generation, the fit becomes somewhat problematic. He is able to speak of "this admirable *machine* and frame of man's body"
because no internal force, spirit, or agent has guided its construction, but the
very language that asserts the deterministic force of the mechanistic process simultaneously and paradoxically gives volition to the "machine" (*TT*, 231). The rhetorical question "can it choose but to" is an oxymoron; whatever the delimitations
on its range of options, the "machine" of conception is posited as an agent that
makes a choice. The repeated oxymoron in fact registers precisely the issue that
troubles the theory: does generation result in an automaton driven by necessity
or in a volitional agent?

A similarly telling rhetorical slippage emerges in Digby's record of his observation of the process of chick development, where the chick embryo/fetus is
treated as both a passive object acted upon by forces external to it and as a living, volitional being.[39] He writes:

you may lay severall egges to hatch; and by breaking them at severall ages you may
distinctly observe every hourely mutation in them, if you please. The first will bee, that
on one side you shall find a great resplendent clearnesse in the white. After a while, a
litle spott of red matter like bload, will appeare in the middest of that clearnesse fas-

tened to the yolke . . . From this red specke, after a while there will streame out, a number of litle (almost imperceptible) red veines. Att the end of some of which, in time there will be gathered together, a knotte of matter which by litle and litle, will take the form of a head . . . But by litle and litle the rest of the body of an animal is framed out of those red veines which streame out all aboute from the hart. And in process of time, that body incloseth the heart within it by the chest. . . . After which this litle creature soone filleth the shell, by converting into severall partes of it self all the substance of the egge. And then growing weary of so straight an habitation, it breaketh prison, and cometh out, a perfectly formed chicken.( *TT*, 220–21)

In the first section of this description, the observer is by and large the grammatical subject. Digby wants to tell his readers what they will see if they repeat his labors, so he allows them vicariously to observe for themselves the emergence of the chick through his detailed description. The repeated phrases what "you shall find," what "you will ere long beginne to discerne" or "may distinctly observe" both bring the reader imaginatively into the arena of inspection and reinforce his sense of his subject status in the process. During this part of the passage, the chick is the grammatical object, merely a little spot of red matter like blood that "is so litle, that you can not see it, but by the motion of it." In the second section, the embryo becomes the grammatical subject, but the verbs are all passive: a "knotte" "will be gathered together"; "the rest of the body of an animal is framed out" until the body closes over the heart. The body here seems to be developing by means of external, unnamed powers; it is functioning like a machine, without recourse to "a cunning artificer." In the last few lines, however, the subject suddenly shifts to the chick itself, now conceived of as a little creature endowed with the power to "convert" matter into itself, subject to moods that compel it to "break" from its "prison," and granted the ability to "come . . . out, a perfectly formed chicken."

This grammatical transference enacts the same sleight of hand presented by the bean that cannot but choose to become a plant. A mechanical theory of generation that posits the actual production of parts cannot account for the generation of volitional beings. Rhetoric, therefore, accomplishes the work that theory cannot perform on its own; it simply grants subjectivity to the creature once it has developed and grown to a "perfect" point.

Digby's theory did not attract many followers, any more than had Descartes's similar attempt at mechanical epigenesis (written several years earlier, it was not published until 1662).[40] One problem besetting mechanical epigenesis was

how to explain the structural complexity of living organisms; physical proper-
ties like density and rarity did not of themselves seem able to account for the
emergence of the high degree of complexity that microscopists were then discovering in even the tiniest of creatures. Furthermore, short of calling upon an
act of Providence in each instance of creation (which Digby, for one, explicitly
denied), mechanism could not sufficiently account for the emergence of life from
inanimate matter (see *TT*, 227). Later in the century, Bernard de Fontenelle made
a joke about mechanical explanations of physiology altogether: "Do you say that
beasts are machines just as watches are? Put a male dog-machine and a female
dog-machine side by side, and eventually a third little machine will be the result,
whereas two watches will lie side by side all their lives without ever producing
a third watch."[41]

Responding in part to these issues, the theories offered by Nathaniel Highmore and William Harvey were explicitly vitalist.[42] Harvey and Highmore, who
each published their work on generation about seven years after Digby, differed
on the manner of embryogeny itself, but in determining a cause for the evident
complexity of living things, both invoked precisely what Digby had sought to
avoid: a "cunning artificer" who guides the process of generation. For Harvey,
as we saw, the embryo is responsible for its own growth and development, and
it is directed by a vital spirit that is innate to it; for Highmore, the spiritual form,
or what he calls "the soul playing the skilful Workman," is transferred to the
embryo through the father's semen and is therefore able to direct its progress.[43]
Highmore clearly states that it is the soul that actually generates the new being
when he insists that generation occurs *only* when the soul decides to accompany
the sperm in its venture. When the father's soul becomes "intent on propagation and multiplying her self into another Individuum," Highmore explains, she
"diffuseth her self into the . . . parting sperm" and makes them "prolifical":

> Which coming into a convenient receptacle, where these Atomes may repose; being
> moved onely by that soul which accompanied them, and from which they received
> their orders and commands, are soon setled into their proper places, and become a
> perfect *Individuum of that Species*. (*HG*, 111; emphasis mine)[44]

Highmore's reliance on the father's soul as a "skilful Workman" allows him to
counter Digby's inability to explain sufficiently the cause of complexity and variety. Highmore had rejected Digby's theory precisely because the "accidental and
equivocal parents" of heat and cold, density and rarity, could not of themselves

constitute the "fruitful Mother of this variety" (*HG*, 14, 18). But implicitly, High-more's vitalist explanation also counters the absence of a source of distinctive human identity in Digby's theory because he provides for the genealogical trans-ference of the formative soul from the father to the fetus through the father's semen; the father's semen moved by the father's soul makes the individual.

It seems apparent then that the problems posed by mechanical epigenesis concerned more than issues of structural complexity and divine intervention in generation. At stake as well was the distinctiveness of *human* generation and therefore of human identity, since if one does not admit divine intervention in the generation of each living being, what is there to distinguish the birth of a man from the emergence of a crystal other than mere physical structure, or from a bean that cannot choose but to become a plant? Harvey's and Highmore's responses at least had the advantage of being able to posit identity through the efficacy of a vital spirit, whether that derive from an external source (as in High-more) or be inherent to the creature itself (as in Harvey).

Also at issue in these theories was the question of paternal agency in the gen-eration of identity. Whereas Highmore asserted the traditional claim of the father's primacy in transferring the formative soul that determines the organism's *telos*, Digby and Harvey challenged it—the former by claiming the deterministic nature of development, the latter by claiming that the animating spirit is inherent to the organism itself. Given their implications for questions of paternal or patri-archal primacy in the construction of identity, it is not surprising that these the-ories arose in England at just the time when the status of political identity was a topic of revolution—that is, between 1644, when Digby's *Two Treatises* was pub-lished, and 1651, when Harvey and Highmore published. In the transition from contested monarchy to Commonwealth and reverberating from the moment of the regicide was the question of the continued viability of the old idea of the King as God's stepstool and thereby as the only source of political identity and obligation. As I argued in the last chapter, one way to understand the emer-gence of these particular embryological theories at precisely the moment when that idea was under extreme pressure is to see them in relation to the question of political identity being posed at the time. Considered in its broader cultural context, Highmore's reliance on the paternal soul that grants identity to the embryo through the aegis of the male semen affords a physiological analog to the genetic argument of political patriarchy in which one's identity in the fam-ily and State is determined by the father, or, more broadly, by the King. By contrast, Harvey's revolutionary understanding of the artificer as inherent to the creature itself evokes within the domain of the body the emergence of the self-determining citizen within the public realm.[45] These biological theories, in other words, at least implicitly take part in the contemporary debate about whether identity, physiological or political, can emerge from a source other than the patriarch.

Historians of science have suggested that the particular theories propounded by Digby, Harvey, and Highmore did not take hold in the later seventeenth century for readily apparent reasons: on the one side, Digby's mechanical epigenesis simply did not work, and, on the other side, Harvey's and Highmore's vitalist theories were couched in a language of spiritual form and formative virtue that was on the wane. Understood in these terms, the emergence of more mechanistic models of generation that arose in the 1660s and after accords with the field's internal logic; a theory was needed that would cohere more nearly with the reigning mechanistic thinking of the time and that did not have to make thorny theological claims about the emergence of life from inanimate matter.[46]

The mechanistic models of embryonic growth offered in the metamorphosis and preformation theories of the late seventeenth century filled both these requirements, though, as some have noted, more by resituating than resolving the problem of how life actually is generated.[47] But given the embeddedness of theories of embryology in cultural concerns about the origins and nature of identity, it seems perfectly consistent that as the experiment in revolution gave way to a return to monarchy, these earlier theories would be no longer resonant—because they throw into relief the question of the source of identity and raise the possibility that it lies someplace other than with the traditional patriarchy.[48] Whatever the cause, the shift to more mechanistic models of embryogeny exerted new pressures on the notion of the self, and, as if in compensatory response, a newly characterized embryo emerged; unlike the theories that preceded them, both metamorphosis and preformation theory were adamant in their assertions of the unchanging identity of the products of generation.

In suggesting that the whole child exists just a few days after conception, Kerckring was supporting the theory of metamorphosis, the first of the mechanistic theories that gained prominence in the second half of the seventeenth century. The theory had several variations, but the general idea was that some time after fecundation, either the whole organism or at least the rudiments of the whole organism emerge simultaneously rather than sequentially, as epigenetic theories had proposed. Unlike epigenesis, metamorphosis denies the production of anything substantially new after conception and posits instead the steady enlargement of parts already present (though not necessarily visible) from the first. Rather than explain the actual creation of new parts of a living organism, metamorphosis explained generation as a matter of mechanical growth of parts already there; not so much concerned with parental contributions or with embryogenesis itself, it concentrates instead on the emergence of the embryo once fertilization has occurred and on the embryo's subsequent growth. The theory was quite popular in the second half of the seventeenth century, and it was supported in various forms by Henry Power, Anthony Everard, and Marcello Malpighi, among others.

The work of Dr. William Croone, who read a paper on generation to the Royal Society in 1671, demonstrates how the claim of mechanical generation in animals is offset by the more urgent claim that the organism produced has an immediately recognizable and stable identity.[49] In a paper presented as a personal essay, Croone announces his discovery that "the body of the chick is formed at the very moment of conception," and "perchance . . . even before it has left the hen's body" (*OG*, 117, 125). Croone makes a minimal gesture toward individuating his embryos by claiming that they grow at their own idiosyncratic rates, but he asserts that they come into being "entire at one stroke" as if from a "mould" (*OG*, 112). Precisely because the report is written as a personal narrative, complete with details of his mistakes and wrong turns, it becomes fairly evident that Croone was determined to find evidence of metamorphosis in his research, regardless of what he claims he actually saw, as if in blind determination to discover a whole being at the very start of generation. This is especially apparent in the story he tells of his accidental discovery of the chick miniature: Croone explains that when he returned to a newly-laid egg that he had recently placed by a hearth, he saw that part of the yolk had begun to grow hard. After removing the hardened bits and giving over the rest of the egg to a servant "to cook for household purposes," Croone almost absentmindedly threw into a dish of warm water "the particle of yolk . . . encrusted by the heat of the fire and still hanging from the scissors" (*OG*, 120). Presently, he says, "a hard skin like a very faint mist" separated off from the rest of the piece of yolk. Slowly, this skin unfolded and, as he watched intently, Croone says, "I *seemed to see* something very like the head of an embryo or chick." Next, he says, he "scanned with eager eyes all there was to see, and *observed quite clearly and distinctly*" the eyes and beak, the ribs, the feet, and even the umbilical vessels (*OG*, 121; emphasis mine). Croone moves from possibility to certainty, from what "seemed" to be the case to what was quite clear and distinct, without a conceptual segue, so that, when he makes the astonishing announcement that he "can . . . *confidently claim* . . . that none of those primordia or evidences of a future chick . . . appear without the whole chick being already present at the same time" (*OG*, 125), the statement has the force of self-evidence.

Croone's willingness to see the complete embryo in an unincubated egg has been explained by his unwitting hardening of a piece of the vitelline membrane, which unfortunately took on the vague characteristics of a chick embryo as it solidified near the fire.[50] But that Croone warns that it will be difficult to replicate his results because, as he readily acknowledges, it is rather hard to find a complete miniature in an unincubated egg surely suggests that his desires constrained his observations. Somehow, it was important for him, as it was for Kerckring as well, to assert the immediate identity of the embryo from its first appearance.

To get a sense of what is at stake in terms of identity formation here, it is important to recall the ways in which the metamorphic embryo differs from earlier versions of the epigenetic embryo that these researchers were trying to discount. Harvey had coined the term "epigenesis" to describe the process of generation by which the parts of the embryo are produced and grow sequentially, a process that begins with an undifferentiated speck of material and ends with a complexly organized, full-grown fetus. Aristotle, also an epigenecist, believed that the semen provided the *telos* of the future embryo by transferring to the female contamena the ability to differentiate and grow. For Aristotle, therefore, the power to become a fetus is derivative; the embryo is made only by the power of the semen directing it.

Although Harvey followed Aristotle in much else, he argued against Aristotle that the power to grow and differentiate was inherent to the embryo itself. Harvey's embryo, we remember, is thus truly self-made, in that it directs its own transformation from a homogeneous mass to a heterogeneous complexity. However, this characterization of the embryo as a self-directing subject is not applied from the first; in its earliest stages, the ovum or primordium has life only in potentia and the substance that appears on the twenty-first day after coitus Harvey calls an "unshapen Worme or Maggot" (*DG*, 415). So it is pretty clear that however Harvey subjectified the fetus, the earliest stages of the embryo more nearly resemble vegetable or vermicular life than they do animal or human.

The metamorphic embryo, by contrast, does not *become* an animal or a human fetus; it already is that from the start. Identity is not something that is self-created or that develops over time; it is given at conception and then remains stable throughout the growth process. Compared to the embryos of epigenesis, which call into question the existence and source of identity, the metamorphic embryo asserts its identity unambiguously. What it lacks, however, is any clear sense of individuation or agency, in other words, of subjectivity. That this step was taken by preformation theory (in one of its forms) suggests a specific correlation between mechanism and subject status: the more indebted a theory is to mechanical explanation, the more the need to assert the subjectivity of its products.

. Preformation theory, which gained currency toward the end of the century, is similar to metamorphosis in that both theories assume the simultaneous appearance of all parts (or all important parts) of the embryo. But whereas metamorphosis asserts that the embryo suddenly crystallizes some time after conception, and thus assumes that fertilization actually creates the embryo, preformation posits the rudiments of the complete organism in the pregenerative germ, that is, in either the egg or (what we call) the sperm alone. Preformation thus pushes back the reach of mechanism in the process of what now may rightly be called reproduction. Metamorphosis does not explain it, but it does assume the emergence of complexity from some act of generation. Preformation, by contrast, never really permits an act of generation at all: no being is *created* through the interaction of male and female parts; rather, the beings are always in some sense already there, virtually embedded in a single parent's germ.[51] Reproduction itself therefore involves only the unfolding and enlarging of already existent parts, and the purpose of coitus is either, in the ovist version of the theory, for the sperm to activate the embryo's growth in the egg or, in the spermaticist version, for the animalcule to find an appropriate nidus or egg in which to grow.

Preformation was given a good deal of credence by Jan Swammerdam's work during the last decades of the century. In 1670, *Philosophical Transactions* reported that Swammerdam had been able "to shew all the parts of the Butterfly in a Caterpillar" and therefore to demonstrate that "the caterpillar is the butterfly itself, only covered over with a mantle."[52] Swammerdam's findings were tremendously important because they offered physical evidence that animals could exist in miniature before they were large enough to be visible. On this basis, Swammerdam premised at least the plausibility of preformation: if the incipient parts of a butterfly exist in the caterpillar, then why not the incipient parts of other creatures inside unfertilized eggs?[53] Swammerdam believed that an egg is an already living entity containing all the rudiments of the future organism and that the function of the semen is therefore to spark the entity to grow. His conclusion from this marks the beginnings of a thoroughly new understanding of the generative process: "there is no Generation in Nature," he says, " but only a production of growing parts."[54] Although by claiming that the egg is already in some sense alive Swammerdam admits some element of vitalism into his theory, he does not explain how the preformed egg itself is formed; the explanatory range of his theory is therefore thoroughly mechanical.[55] Generation as such is denied, and in its stead emerges a process that literally *re-produces* in elaborated form what already somehow exists in the parental germ.

But simultaneously with preformation's denial of generation and generative agency, there is an insistence that the personhood of the creature comes to be at an ever earlier stage, for now the miniature can be said to exist in some sense even before fecundation. Importantly, however, the two versions of preformationist theory that were most frequently debated in the last quarter of the seventeenth century do not mete out the personhood of the embryo or prefertilized germ equally to the two sexes. Even though the logic of preformation theory should grant the same kind of subject status to the preformed miniature in both its ovist and animalculist versions, it is only the latter that insistently subjectifies the miniature in its rhetoric: the egg, even when it alone houses the rudiments of the complete organism, is rhetorically figured as passive, even if alive. It is this asymmetry that will be most telling about what is at stake in the mechanization of embryology theories and, perhaps, in the mechanization of the world picture at large.

Consider, for example, an anonymous letter to the Royal Society printed in 1683, in which a physician and Fellow of the Royal Society recounts his dissection of a bitch to demonstrate the veracity of the ovist version of preformation. The dog had died from an abdominal pregnancy caused by a blockage in her "uterine horns"; the doctor reasons that organisms must come from eggs alone because there was clearly no room for the semen to pass through the "horns" to get to the egg. Thus he concludes that in the eggs of animals, "the Parts of the Embryo are designed and drawn out, before the Eg has been at all affected by the Masculine Seed."[56] In ovist preformation, therefore, the miniature exists in some sense even before the egg is fertilized, presumably by some form of "irradiation" or vaporous action. But neither the ovum nor the maternal body directs the patterning; the parts of the embryo are "drawn out," "designed" by some unnamed power.

Given passive language such as this, it becomes hard to accept the arguments offered by some historians that ovism presented a brief moment of female empowerment in the history of early modern embryology.[57] In fact, after the work of de Graaf and others had demonstrated what was taken to be the existence of eggs in quadrupeds, ovists generally assumed that fertilization occurred not by material contact between the ovum and the animalcule but, rather, by means of the semen's refined and ethereal nature.[58] As Edward Ruestow explains, "the impregnating principle of the semen was variously described as spirit, vapor, odor, or 'irradiation.'"[59] Thus, even in a theory that offers the female as the origin of the complete miniature, the male role is characterized not as a mechanical trigger but as a spiritual and primary force.

The passive construction of an embryo whose parts "are designed and drawn out" also suggests another of the attractions of mechanical explanation in preformation theory, namely, that it left room for a higher power in the reproductive process. Since preformation accounts only for the growth of already existent parts (generally remaining silent on the question of how the preformed germs actually get preformed), all true generation is at least implicitly left to God.[60] Attributing actual creation to God ensures both that the theory will not be rejected as atheist (a response met, for example, by Digby's proposals) and that mechanical forces do not have to be responsible for generating life. More subtly, however, the implicit move to a supernatural source of creation enforces a boundary between the self, or identity, governed by God, and bodily structures, which function as physiological machines.

And yet it was just that divide that kept threatening to collapse as the penchant for mechanizing various physiological processes, now including generation, continued to thrive in the late seventeenth century. The enthusiasm for mechanism, in fact, led to an often explicit anxiety about what that meant for man's integrity as a human being, as if the marvel of man's mechanized body might also entail a similarly mechanized self. The Cambridge Platonist Ralph Cudworth, for example, worried that Hobbes's reduction of all mental processes to matter and motion suggested that men themselves were "really Nothing else, but Machines, and Automata."[61] Humphrey Ditton was more pointed in his concern: mechanic thinkers, he complained, "have made the whole Universe a meer Lump of Matter; and Man, the most elegant and lovely Creature of all, they have complimented no higher, than to given him the Title of the best and finest Piece of Clock-work . . . so that we are only a Set of Moving pratling Machines."[62] The mechanization of the body, it seems, threatened to rob man of his identity as a volitional agent. If generation proceeds like "clock-work"—we can recall here the threatened uniformity of Croone's embryos that arise as if from being stamped in a mold—if man does not ever really create, but rather only re-produces what is already there, without self-determination and self-direction, how is man different from a machine built invariably to churn out its products?

That the ovist model in the seventeenth century made passive objects of both the mother and the ovum suggests that the mechanization of the female body was not seen as problematic at the time. By the mid-eighteenth century, however, this was no longer true; as Andrea Henderson has argued, preformation theories gradually fell out of favor in the late eighteenth century in part because the tendency "to make mothers appear to be machines and babies to be little more than commodities became increasingly intolerable," largely because it "made the mother appear to stand in a relation of ownership to the child."[63] But Henderson's observations about the fetus as a product of its mother's labor are applicable only to the ovist version of preformation; animalculism always resisted such objectification.

This becomes apparent in Dr. George Garden's brief survey of seventeenth-century embryology, "A Discourse Concerning the Modern Theory of Generation," printed in *Philosophical Transactions* in 1691.[64] In describing what he considers to be the outmoded ovist view of generation, Garden continues to treat the maternal body and the egg itself as passive objects but suggests a creative agency in the activity of the sperm. He explains that though "the rudiments of each animal were originally [thought to reside] in the respective females," it was the males' "spirituous liquor" that would "insinuate its self" into the "Ducts and Pores of the Rudiments of those Animals which were in greatest forwardness in the Ovary" and that would thereby "extend and enlarge all their parts, and at last bring them to perfection."[65] Though he is describing ovist preformation, Garden nonetheless traces all the productive responsibility to the male's contribution: both mother and miniature are passive recipients of the male's "spirituous" power.

When Garden next describes the new animalculist version, which he endorses, suddenly the miniature is given an active role while the mother remains passive:

> It is acknowledged by all, that the *foetus in utero* for some considerable time after conception has no connexion with the womb, that it sits wholly loose to it, and is perfectly a little round egg with the foetus in its midst, which sends forth its umbilical vessels by degrees, and at last lays hold on the uterus.[66]

Formed in the father, the entity is instantly deemed a fetus at conception and immediately takes responsibility for its growth. Not the recipient of nurturing care, and dependent on the maternal body only to the extent that it can claim

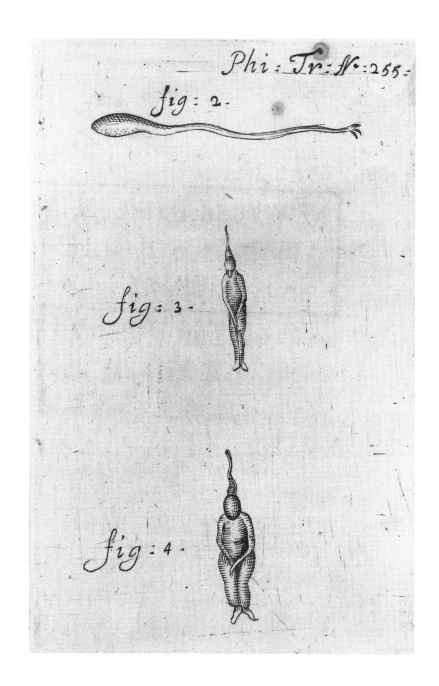

*Plate 10. From* Philosophical Transactions of the Royal Society *(London, 1699), the plate depicts sperm shaped as miniature men.*

it for its use, the fetus is a conqueror who sends forth its "vessels" and "lays hold" on its newfound territory. That territory, of course, is the female reproductive body, which Garden's language casts as unrelated to the newly emerged being. Thus, of the three terms he uses to denote the female organ that houses the fetus ("*in utero*," "womb," and "uterus"), the vernacular term, and therefore the term that arguably is the most evocative of the woman's body, the "womb," appears only in the context of denying any connection between it and the fetus; the fetus exists "*in utero*" and lays hold of "the uterus," but has "no connexion" with "the womb."

Garden's rhetoric of territorial conquest is apparent also in Anton von Leeu-wenhoeck's correspondence with the Royal Society during the last quarter of the seventeenth century. Leeuwenhoeck first reported to the Royal Society his finding of "little animals in the semen" in the late 1670s; over the next few decades, he increasingly urged on a reluctant audience his belief that the sperm alone carried the miniature of the future organism. In doing so, Leeuwenhoeck fre-quently made the sperm itself, and not just the embryo it becomes, a little man, an adventurer on rough seas. In explaining, for example, why there should be in semen so many animalcules if only one is needed for generation, Leeuwen-hoeck stages a little drama: "in the Womb," he says,

> each Animalcule might suffice for a Generation, if the place where it comes to be nursed be fit for it; But the womb being so large in Comparison of so small a crea-ture, and there being so few Vessels and places fit to see it . . . there cannot be too great a number of Adventurers, when there is so great a likelihood to miscarry.[67]

For Leeuwenhoeck, the animalcule, which alone carries the rudiments of the future organism, is a daring adventurer, traveling through the perils of an over-whelming womb, seeking to find its proper resting spot.

Admittedly, Leeuwenhoeck's rhetoric is usually not this florid; in fact, the translated excerpts from his letters published in *Philosophical Transactions* are known for their straightforward, non-metaphoric style. Yet he consistently thought of the sperm as little animals, as active, striving, goal-oriented entities, even when he would claim with certainty only that they could form a child not that they were themselves little children.[68] From this perspective, the famous hoax in which the pseudonymous "Dalenpatius" claimed actually to *see* the minia-ture in the sperm is simply a logical extension of what the rhetoric of animal-culist preformation already implied: though the process of reproduction is mechanical, the preformed miniature constitutes an active agency, even within the body of the father (plate 10).[69]

There seems, then, to be an important asymmetry between the ovist and the animalculist versions of preformation theory; for both, the maternal body is a passive receptacle, useful only as the place in which the embryo may arrange its growth. But whereas in the ovist version, the miniature is also passive, acted upon by powers outside the explanatory range of the theory, in the animalculist version, the embryo itself is rhetorically empowered to direct its course. Perhaps one explanation for the asymmetry is that some (including Leeuwenhoeck) thought that the animalcules were themselves animals, that is, microscopic organisms living in the semen just as there were now demonstrated to be microscopic organisms living within tiny drops of pond water. If animalcules were actually animals, then it would be fitting to characterize them as purposive agents.

But the differing rhetoric of ovist and animalculist description suggests that something more is at work here. If the maternal body were to be the sole provider of the future organism, it was somehow permissible, at least at first, to think of it as a machine, a living object acted on by forces beyond its control. But if the only true parent were the father, if the sperm contained all the ingredients for the future being, then that being could not be thought of as a machine, because the father could not be thought of in those terms. The only way to protect the integrity of adult masculine subjectivity in the face of a mechanistic theory that would rob men of it was to inscribe that subjectivity onto the seed that becomes the man. Embryology, in other words, becomes a mode of self-affirmation, and animalculist preformation, finally, not only solves the mystery of generation, by including it under the explanatory umbrella of mechanism, but also alleviates the threat to subjectivity that mechanism so insistently posed.

■ I have tried in this chapter both to document and to account for the emergence of "embryonic individuals" at a time when what we generally think of as "early modern identity" was first being fashioned. I have argued that these embryonic individuals in their various forms arose partly as a result of a shift in the way embryological research was materially practiced but also, and more radically, as a result of ideological threats to subjectivity posed by the increasing reliance on mechanism in the theories themselves. If this argument suggests something about embryology, that it needs to be read symptomatically, that its rhetoric is necessarily a register of the culture in which it functions, it also suggests something about the construction of early modern identity itself—that its distinguishing features of autonomy and self-determination arise not so much as unencumbered achievements of human reason or human will, but rather as compensatory responses to perceived threats to the unique and privileged status of human, and particularly masculine, identity. The more man in his physiology resembles a machine or the product of a machine (something stamped in a mold), the more it becomes necessary to ensure that he is known to be something other than a machine—that he is a person, a human, a subject, from the first moment of his conception, or even before.

# 6 / The Masculine Subject of Touch:

## Case Histories from the Birthing Room

I N  H I S  1 7 3 3  *E S S A Y  O N  T H E  I M P R O V E M E N T  O F  M I D -
wifery*, the London surgeon Edmund Chapman tells the story of a "poor
unhappy woman" who had been plagued by violent, periodic pains in her
belly and back for seven days. She was attended by "several persons of an
inferior Class in the Practice of Physick" as well as by a number of midwives,
but everyone, including the woman herself, was, Chapman says, "confounded,
and at a loss," unable to make sense of her condition.[1] When at last he was called,
Chapman sent out all but a few of the "numerous company" that had gathered
about the patient and then proceeded to establish the following information
through a remarkable physical exam:

> Where the Rima Magna should have been there was only the Appearance of a
> small Slit or Aperture. . . . Nor was there the least Sign of the Clitoris or Nymphae
> to be seen or felt. This imperfect vagina, or rather slit, before mentioned, was just big
> enough to receive one Finger, with which I endeavoured to find out the Mouth of the
> Womb, but in vain; for on the Hinder-part, or towards the Os Sacrum, there was no
> passage at all, whilst Forwards, and under the Os Pubis, it admitted my Finger without
> much Resistance. At this Part, (which was also very dry,) there was not the least Force,
> Pain, or Swelling; whilst wholly Backwards, at the Anus, there were all. The Anus was
> dilated to a great degree, (even enough to receive my Hand,) tho' very thick and much
> swelled quite round. In that Part too there was a large Tumour which bore hard down,
> and even out of the Body at every Pain. (*IM*, 88–89)

By performing his manual maneuvers, Chapman realized that the woman's distended intestine harbored a child pressing to be born. After allowing the mid-

wives to "see and feel how all things were," Chapman made an aperture with his lancet, dilated the orifice with his fingers and delivered the woman "of a child at the anus." The "unfortunate woman," subject of this "strange and unnatural" case, he tells his readers, was "quite spent, before I was called in"; she lived two or three days, and then she died. In closing, however, Chapman suggests knowingly that "she might have been saved, had the Operation been performed sooner, and in time" (*IM*, 90).

Chapman clearly has some lessons to teach with this "strange and unnatural" case, the most obvious among them, the need to call for appropriate help in a timely manner and the importance of surgical intervention in certain medical contexts. But surely more is going on here. Told in the first person, the narrative allows Chapman to construct himself as the solitary authority in an otherwise communal endeavor. Where the "numerous" others gathered in the birthing room display dangerous ignorance, Chapman achieves an unequivocal certainty about the woman's condition. By touching her inside and out, Chapman establishes precise and exclusive knowledge both of her strange anatomy and of what is going on inside it. Through his deliberate, masterful manual examination, through the conclusion he thereby draws and the actions he thereafter takes, Chapman emerges in the case as the epitome of early modern man—rational, knowledgeable, measured, efficient, and singularly authoritative. Any trace of irrationality, any hint of ignorance or chaos, is displaced onto the community of others in the room who do not know what to do, and onto the "strange and unnatural" body of the woman herself. Chapman's self-construction transpires therefore through two different though related imputed oppositions: one between himself and the other assembled practitioners, the other between himself and the woman he treats. He defines himself by way of a series of contrasts— his singularity against the midwives' community, his rationality against their ignorance, his expertise against the woman's helpless suffering.

And yet these oppositions are not easy or exact. As a surgeon, Chapman himself might very well be considered of an inferior class in the practice of medicine precisely because surgeons, unlike physicians, engaged in the messy manual labor of handling and cutting the body, and here Chapman engages in a rather aggressive mode of such labor. But far from acknowledging any illicit or erotic associations of his extensive manual penetrations, his finger in her slit, his hand up her anus, Chapman presents himself instead as a paradigm of decorous rationality. The case history thus offers more than the details of one unfortunate woman's demise; we watch a kind of transformation, or, more exactly, a self-construction by way of transformation, as Chapman converts his manual ministrations into a vehicle of his rationality, his affiliation with the unnatural body of a woman into a means of asserting his knowing mastery over and above it. If Chapman comes off here as a model of early modern subjectivity, it is a model uneasily erected on vexed opposition.

Chapman's case history, and the others like it we will examine in this chapter, marks a final transition in our study from a focus on the body abstractly conceived to specific instances of embodiment. My concern so far has been to trace out the assumptions of and implications for personhood in rhetorical formulations of the body as it was philosophically, physiologically, and therapeutically conceived. But amid all the diversity of the texts so far considered, the focus was on the body as an abstraction, an idea, a generic norm, and thereby as a record of inscribing precepts of personhood in early modern culture. In this chapter I want to look at particular bodies as they are represented in case histories, the stories of individual practitioners and their patients. As we saw briefly with Chapman, questions of personhood still pertain but the overall concerns are somewhat different. How are we to understand the proliferation of midwifery books generally and midwifery case histories specifically in the context of the competitive and changing "medical marketplace" of late seventeenth- and early eighteenth-century England? Are they simply what they purport to be, namely, educative manuals for the professional and lay public? And how do the new realities of medical practice—specifically, the entry of men into midwifery and the innovative techniques for delivering babies they brought with them—impinge on questions of personhood, both for practitioners and patients?[2]

Until the late seventeenth century, English midwifery texts were largely unoriginal, being mostly translations and compilations of Latin and Continental sources. They were furthermore written didactically, giving putative instruction on what one was to do in any given circumstance, rather than recounting what the practitioner did him- or herself. But by the end of the seventeenth century, a new kind of midwifery text began to appear, both in manuscript and in printed form, which focused on the particular experiences of individual practitioners. These are among the first collections of medical case histories in English, and they differed from their predecessors both in being largely original and in their focused attention to the character and accomplishments of the practitioners who wrote them.

The practitioners portrayed in these self-authored case histories all advertise new techniques for touching the parturient body, either directly, through the manual manipulation of the fetus or the mother, or indirectly, through the use of instruments like the forceps and the fillet. They thus routinely and palpably engage their patients' bodies, touching, penetrating, manipulating them to ease delivery. And they are also fully cognizant of the somatic experience of those they treat, the dangers childbirth poses, the pain it routinely entails. In these narrative accounts, much of this somatic experience (for both practitioner and patient) gets rendered in acute detail precisely because the practitioner is so thoroughly "in touch" with the patient's body; the practitioner feels, literally, sensibly, the state of the childbearing woman.

And yet it is the practitioner's bodily touch that paradoxically becomes the vehicle for the body's transcendence. These case histories thus offer concrete instances of what we have seen more abstractly in bio-medical writing throughout the period: the consolidation of a subject gendered as masculine, a subject that is autonomous, authoritative, self-directing, and, above all, distinct from the body, by at once engaging and superceding what gets marked as material or (merely) embodied. These case histories demonstrate the consolidation of authoritative, autonomous, mind-defined subjects, but not in isolation, not in relation only to themselves; they must enlist what they cast as their opposites in order to distinguish themselves as singular. This ground-against-which has at least two facets here; on the one hand, the competing practitioners of the marketplace and, on the other, the patient the author treats. And yet, as we saw with Chapman, the opposition is never neat because the practitioners themselves use manual techniques that threaten to associate them with manual (as opposed to rational) labor, and because the patient is ever present to the practitioner as a participatory subject in the process of childbirth. What we will find, therefore, in the generation of the masculine subject of childbirth, is a reconfiguration both of the "handiwork" of midwifery and of the status of the women literally handled. This process in the end does not deny the body; rather, it enlists the body to demonstrate its subjugation, thereby to assert the modern transcendence of masculine mind.

■ The often rehearsed story of the entrance of men into the routine practice of midwifery in the late seventeenth and early eighteenth centuries has historically been somewhat of a didactic affair, its older versions typically resembling morality tales more than reasoned analysis. The stories tend to take one of two opposing forms: in the early histories of obstetrics starting in the late nineteenth century, the medical men are portrayed as being educated and compassionate, and their eventual triumph over ignorant, intrusive midwives is understood exclusively as evidence of the medical Enlightenment.[3] After the 1960s, when women began to write about the topic, the men become self-serving and avaricious, wielding instruments as weapons, and their forcible ejection of capable women from the only profession in which they had historically held a monopoly is understood as an instance of women's social oppression.[4] Assessing the history of the debate, Lisa Cody neatly encapsulates its opposing evaluative terms: the emergence of male midwives is an example of either "medical glory" or "gory misogyny."[5]

If in recent years this debate has become somewhat less of an exercise in polemic, its assumption that competition between the sexes drives the story of early-modern midwifery and should therefore drive its analysis has not dramatically changed. Adrian Wilson, for example, has argued that male midwifery could have succeeded only if women wanted it to, since it was typically women who determined whom to call to their deliveries and when.[6] Wilson's claim that childbirth was "still a collective female affair" even as men overtook the profession adds nuance to the story, but the story is still primarily about the interplay of social-sexual roles.[7] Even as careful a scholar as Doreen Evenden is willing to caricature the efforts of the eighteenth-century male midwife: "By the 1750s," she says, "midwives' traditional, practical skill proved no match for the claims of the male midwife, waiting in the wings with his shiny instruments and promises of 'scientific expertise.'"[8] Much modern scholarship seems to replicate the gender conflict that underlies the history it studies; male scholars analyze with varying degrees of approval the emergence of male midwifery, while women scholars analyze the same set of circumstances with varying levels of disdain.

To be sure, there is ample reason to read the story of the shifts in early modern midwifery practice precisely this way, in terms of the gender divide between male and female practitioners. Jane Sharp, who in 1671 was the first woman to publish a midwifery manual in English, explicitly addressed her guide to her "sisters," the "midwives of England," and, while she "cannot deny, that men in some things may come to a greater perfection of knowledge than women ordinarily can," she nonetheless claims women's authority in the birthing room. It is, she says, "the natural propriety of women to be much seeing into that Art."[9] Sarah Stone, writing over sixty years later and the first Englishwoman to write an original midwifery text, similarly speaks to her "sisters in the profession" and rails against the "boyish pretenders" who, she complains, typically enter the birthing room "when the work is near finish'd; and then the Midwife, who has taken all the pains, is accounted of little value, and the young men command all the praise."[10] The works of these midwives attest both to women's articulate awareness of a gender-based shift in their profession and to their ability to combat it with gender-based arguments.

But even if some of the midwifery texts of the period were written as explicit endorsements or rejections of the entrance of men into a traditionally female profession, the gender difference between practitioners is not the only or even the predominant ground of conflict in them. Despite the increasingly vociferous complaints about men in the profession, the majority of midwives even in the 1730s were women, and midwifery books written by both men and women were addressed to women (both female midwives and childbearing women generally) rather than to men (who arguably needed the most instruction, given that they could not have had much experience in attending normal deliveries).[11] And if many of the texts detail the horrors committed by ignorant female midwives, so do many detail the butchery of unskilled men. Although he has much to say against meddlesome midwives, the seventeenth-century physician and male midwife Percival Willughby includes in his *Observations in Midwifery* the story of a gentlewoman who "rotted in the womb" and subsequently died after a "man midwife" inadvertently wounded her with his crochet during a delivery. Willughby complains that "his work was carried on with much unhandsomenes, and accompanied with great ignorance."[12] Similarly, half a century later, Edmund Chapman recounts the story of a male midwife who used the hook to extract a child he had mistakenly taken for dead; when the child emerged from the womb alive, says Chapman, "the wounded infant by its cries and agonies gave much greater pain to the lamenting mother than she had felt before" (*IM*, Preface, n.p.). Stories such as these, written by men about the horrifying errors of men in the birthing room, suggest that to think of the tensions in these texts exclusively in terms of the gender of the practitioners (the men want to oust the women, the women want to ward off the men) is, if clearly not wrong, at least somewhat limiting.

One way to expand an analysis of these midwifery texts is to consider the ways in which they negotiate the tenuous borders dividing medical fields. Traditionally, midwives were called upon to handle all normal deliveries; if a problem arose so that the mother's life was perceived to be in danger and the child was assumed to be dead, say, because of prolonged obstruction or uncontrolled bleeding, a surgeon would be called in to extract the child forcibly (and in pieces, if necessary) with obstetrical instruments such as the hook and crochet (plate

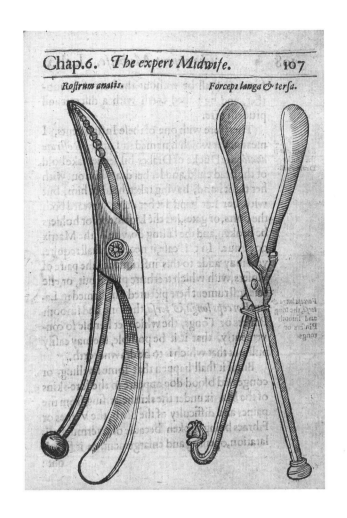

*Plate 11. From Jacob Rueff's* The Expert Midwife *(London, 1637), the plate depicts instruments used for craniotomy.  Reproduced by permission of the Harvey Cushing/John Hay Whitney Medical Library of Yale University.*

11).[13] At least in theory, the roles of midwives and surgeons in the process of child-birth were fairly discrete, and physicians generally were not involved at all. One of the innovations of late seventeenth to early eighteenth-century midwifery was a gradual diluting of this divide among differing types of practitioners. As the position of the so-called man-midwife began to take form, as, that is, physicians began to attend deliveries and surgeons began to attend normal deliveries, the boundaries that distinguished among and therefore defined the different occupations began to give way. If this process promised an expanded arena of medical practice for physicians and surgeons, it also jeopardized the integrity of midwifery as a discrete endeavor. Regarded in this way, the threat posed by the emergence of male midwifery was understood to be a threat to the preserve of midwifery as a distinct profession, at least as much as it was perceived to be an attack on the expertise of women as practitioners.

Jane Sharp's response to this threat is therefore twofold: she is interested in asserting the privileged authority of women *as women* in the birthing room, but, reacting to a perceived effort to break down the boundaries of midwifery from competing practitioners outside her field, Sharp asserts, at least implicitly, the right of midwives to perform the obstetrical functions of surgeons, thereby endeavoring to expand the boundaries of her field from within. Sharp's chapter on "rules for Women that are come to their Labour," for example, is filled with general instructions on how to use "Chirurgeons Instruments" to extract presumably dead fetuses. Yet, oddly for someone presumably seeking to educate, Sharp provides very little actual instruction. Here she describes how to remove a dead fetus that presents feet first:

> If the feet come first fasten the hook upon the bone above the privy parts, called os pubis, or by some rib or back bones, or breast bones; then draw it not forth, but hold the Instrument in your left hand, and then fasten another hook upon some other part of the Child right against the first, and draw gently both together that the Child might come equally, moving it from one side to another until you have drawn it forth altogether; but often guide it with your fore-finger well anointed; if it stick or stop any where, take higher hold still with your hooks upon the dead child.[14]

Surely there is not enough information here actually to teach anyone wielding an instrument. But by its very insufficiency as instruction the passage asserts its unspoken claim that midwives have both the right and the ability to use the instruments of a surgeon. Sharp similarly tells her "sisters" that in certain cases they "must divide the skull and take it out by pieces with instruments for that purpose"; if no midwife could learn by that sentence how to perform a craniotomy, she would at least learn that it is within her province to do so.[15] In devoting the majority of the chapter to the midwife's use of surgical instruments, and yet in not providing any really *useable* information about their employment, Sharp implicitly claims that midwives, regardless of whether they are men or women, can assume the obstetrical work of surgeons.[16]

That such paucity of practical information in early modern midwifery books is not unique to Sharp suggests that, if we want to get a fuller sense of the cultural work they actually performed, we need to look beyond their authors' routine claims that they wrote the books strictly for educative purposes. Doreen Evenden has demonstrated the existence of an elaborate apprenticeship system in London that would have obviated the need for instructional books altogether; considering published material nearly irrelevant for her purposes, Evenden relies exclusively on archival records to reconstruct her picture of seventeenth-century London midwifery. Contemporary writers, even those who published, would probably have agreed with Evenden's conclusions. Sharp introduces herself on the title page of her midwifery manual as a "Practitioner in the Art of Midwifery above thirty years," resting her authority exclusively on her years of practice rather than on any knowledge she gleaned from books. Stone admits that it is not "improper" to read anatomy but, she claims, had she not been instructed by her mother and been her apprentice for six years, "it would have signified little" (*CPM*, xv). Both these writers are pitting their practical experience against book learning in order to establish their authority over the pretensions of Latined men, but for authors of published books to discount the usefulness of books to their practice suggests as well that the work accomplished by those books could not have been purely instructional. Helen King sums up her sense of the midwifery manuals as a group: "Midwives books could . . . be described as a combination of antiquarianism, irrelevance, salaciousness and the blindingly obvious. There is very little on midwifery itself."[17] Though perhaps somewhat of an overstatement, King is surely right to note that these books cannot simply be taken to be historical textbooks, revealing what practitioners actually did.

The work of social and medical historians has thus begun to suggest the need to assess these texts in other ways, pointing us toward the value of reading them not as straightforward registers of historical practice but primarily as rhetorical constructs, as public performances offered for commercial consumption, intended not so much to instruct as to promulgate certain images and identities of the practitioners. That they were essentially commercial ventures more than altruistic efforts in education is repeatedly evident. As we saw in chapter 3, the enormously prolific Nicolas Culpeper characteristically presents himself as a medical reformer struggling against the presumed monopoly on knowledge and medical care possessed by university-trained physicians, but this image must be qualified by his manifest interest in selling lots of books; he routinely refers his readers to the many other books he has written or translated, stressing the importance of his works as a group.[18] Similarly, eighty years later, Chapman announces his wondrous ability to extract obstructed infants alive with the use of the fillet but, it being an instrument of his own invention, he refuses to divulge the details of its construction or the manner of its use (*IM*, 12). Presumably the strategy would encourage women to seek his expertise in their time of labor. These vernacular texts, in other words, were chiefly commercial ventures; whatever actual medical information they conveyed, they functioned rhetorically to construct and commodify a public image of the practitioner of childbirth. That image, I will suggest, epitomizes the modern masculine subject whose generation in the biomedical literature of the time this study has been pursuing.

■ In order to get a sense of the rhetorical effect of a practitioner's touch in the context of childbirth, we need first to get a sense of the nearly complete absence of physical contact in the practice of contemporary medicine generally. As physicians typically performed it in the seventeenth and eighteenth centuries, medical diagnosis made almost no use of physical examination of the patient. Roy Porter describes the typical medical encounter, in which the patient's telling of his or her own history was paramount:

> [The patient] would tell the doctor what was wrong: when and how the complaint had started, what events had precipitated it, the characteristic pains and symptoms, its periodicity. The patient would also describe to his physician key lifestyle features—his eating and sleeping habits, his bowel motions, recent emotional traumas and so forth, not to mention the perhaps slightly indelicate matter of his indulgence in home-made, quack, or patent medicines.[19]

A physician might make some limited physical contact, for example, feeling the pulse to determine its character, and he would make a gross visual assessment of a patient's condition, perhaps noting skin color or the evidence of lesions, but any physical examination was entirely secondary in making a diagnosis to a patient's verbal reporting of his condition.[20] Porter even notes that William Cullen, the top medical practitioner in eighteenth-century Edinburgh, routinely diagnosed his patients by post.[21]

This absence of physical contact between practitioner and patient in the formation of a diagnosis had at least as much to do with an interest in maintaining distinctions among types of practitioners as it did with maintaining norms of modesty. Licensed physicians were university men, trained in the rigors of intellectual labor; it was not within their province to perform manual labor, which was carried out by surgeons.[22] In the highly diversified marketplace of early modern medical practice—a marketplace that included not only physicians, surgeons, and apothecaries, but also midwives, uroscopists, herbalists, empirics, astrologers, lithotomists, and others—a housewife or wise woman of a village might provide care as readily as a licensed physician, and self-diagnosis and self-treatment were not at all uncommon.[23] But given this diversity, or maybe precisely because of it, there was some effort to enforce a divide between those who thought and spoke and those who acted and touched. A physician's physical examination and diagnosis did not become an integral aspect of the medical encounter until the nineteenth century; before that, speech was more important than touch, and it was primarily the speech of the patient that mattered.[24] As W. F. Bynum argues, "the patient's own description of his illness was the pivotal point in the diagnostic process."[25]

It is possible to see this mode of physician–patient interaction in the medical records of Dr. John Symcotts (1592?–1662), who was one of the physicians to Oliver Cromwell and had an extensive practice in Huntingdon and Bedfordshire. The collection of his medical manuscripts (not published until 1951) includes both Symcotts's correspondence with his patients and the casebook he kept of his medical practice from 1636 to 1654. The collection provides some sense of the regularity of self-diagnosis and self-treatment, the absence of any sense of unilateral authority assumed by or accorded to the physician, and the lack of any need for physical examination for accurate (or what was considered accurate) diagnosis. In an anonymous letter from one of his patients, for example, the writer complains:

I have a great burning pain about the reins of my back which strikes up to the very top of my belly, and a wonderful ill scent arising from my stomach. I do desire your best advice. In my hankering for physic I have taken so much all ready and it has done me no good, and therefore I would desire you to send me no physic but some oil or some cooling thing, for I am very sore about my back that I cannot stand upright. The greatest pain of all is my left kidney.[26]

The patient here has both diagnosed and treated himself; he desires the advice of his doctor *by post* but gives no indication that he thinks his doctor's efforts would be compromised by not seeing him. Furthermore, the patient is writing to his doctor, not as a singular medical authority but as another voice in what seems to be a joint effort at analysis.

The casebook as a whole in fact seems generally to be less about Symcotts himself than about ailments and therapies. In contrast to the midwifery case histories, there is only a submerged sense of Symcotts's own subjectivity here. The casebook thus includes many accounts of people cured by non-professionals, like the story of "my lady Cotton," who had "so great a bleeding at the nose that nothing would stay it" but who was then cured by "the cook-maid" after she "took a cloth wet in cold water . . . and made her sit upon it" (*JS*, 71).

It is typical of Symcotts's emphasis on therapy over self-presentation that he includes so many cases that result in death. The following narrative, quoted at length because it so well records his frenetic though ineffective efforts, records the treatments and physical interventions Symcotts offered during the last twenty-four hours of a patient's life:

August 23, 1648. I came to Mr. Egerton, youngest son of the Lord of Bridgwater at Melchburne, who had been about 9 or 10 hours in an apoplexy before I came. I found him in an abolition of all animal functions. His pulse pretty good still and his breathing inequal and interrupted. I caused the smoke of tobacco to be blown up into his nostrils, which he had intermitted; chafed his head with warm cloths, and his neck, crown and ears with the oils of marjoram, sage and amber; put some of them into his mouth and some into his nostrils, which caused his nose to void some drops of blood . . . I caused his hands and feet to be mightily chafed and vehemently struck with our hands, put mustard and vinegar as well as we could into his mouth, blew up sneezing powder . . . which caused him near 20 times to attempt sneezing. Then fomented with the chymical oils again; and caused a hot frying pan to be held close to his head a good while; cupped his shoulders and head without scarification, caused a clyster to be given, which wrought well, then a suppository of alum, which wrought not less. This was iterated to keep the humours in motion. The black plaster was laid to his feet, then pigeons sprinkled with salt; then cupped again and scarified on the shoulders and crown, where, by deep scarification, a vein bled as it had been

from the arm. Leeches were set to the fundament. All in vain, for he died the 24 day
at 12 o'clock at night. (*JS*, 87–88)

Leaving aside the obvious, that it must have been a great relief to all present
that Mr. Egerton was finally released from the misery of medicine, Symcotts himself is a somewhat unstable presence in this case. For the first few sentences, he
speaks in the first person singular, vacillating between what he did himself (I
came, I found, I chafed) and what he caused to be done (smoke to be blown up
his nostrils, hands and feet to be chafed). He seems thus at the start a man of
singular action, making assessments and directing others presumably present.
But as the case progresses, Symcotts recedes as a singular figure through a series
of illogicalities and non-grammaticalities. First he awkwardly aligns the first person singular subject with a first person plural possessive pronoun (I caused his
hands . . . to be . . . struck with our hands); then he commits an illogicality by
combining singular and plural subjects ([I] put mustard and vinegar as well as
we could into his mouth). Rhetorically, the effect of the illogicality is to obscure
Symcotts's distinction as an individuated actor in the sickroom; it becomes impossible to distinguish among things he did alone, caused to be done, and did together
with others. The next sentence omits a subject altogether (Then fomented with
chemical oils again . . .) so that the actions listed only implicitly have agents,
and it is impossible to tell who the agent/s is or are. After that, Symcotts shifts
to the passive voice, taking himself out of the picture altogether (The black plaster was laid to his feet . . .). By the end of the narrative, the dominant impres-
sion left is less of one of a heroic character fighting against the odds as of simply
frantic activity, as one therapy after another is tried and fails. If the patient is
clearly not a subject here, reduced, both by his condition and by the discourse
that describes it, to the etymological meaning of the word, "patient," the one
who suffers, neither is the physician who tries to cure him. The case, in other
words, constructs the practice of medicine (whatever its effects) more clearly
than it constructs medicine's practitioner.

To some extent, the practice of midwifery differed significantly from the practice of other kinds of medicine, for it was always "a work of the Hands," as one
male midwife put it.[27] Midwifery's associations with manual labor are in part
what kept physicians out of the field for so many years; surgeons, who already
worked with their hands, might be called in to take care of obstructed births
with their instruments, but physicians, being thinkers and not touchers, did not
belong here. Yet, even within the context of a profession that required physical

contact, it was a patient's telling of her condition that was paramount. She determined when a child quickened in the womb and she was considered able to inform others whether it had died. So important was the childbearing woman's telling of her body that historians have deemed it more accurate to call her a "participant" rather than a "patient" in the process of birth.[28]

The technical innovations and rediscoveries of seventeenth- and eighteenth-century midwifery that involved the use of touch, such as podalic version, pelvic manipulation, and the use of the forceps and the fillet, changed more than the norms of handling difficult deliveries and the rules for who got to handle them.[29] These shifts in medical practice, as they are recorded in the case histories and treatises of those who promoted them, also produced shifts in the self-presentation of the practitioners and in their constructed connection to others engaged in the birthing process. Whatever the historical reality of the relative authority and engagement of the people involved in the birthing process, the childbearing woman is decreasingly present as a subject in these texts. Her verbal participation becomes either irrelevant or obviated altogether; gossips and competing practitioners, be they other midwives or physicians called in before the author's arrival, are similarly constructed as backdrop to the author's more elaborate self-construction. Advocating the advantages of physical contact and yet seeking to establish their rational authority, practitioners had to counter the cultural norms that aligned touch at best with manual labor and at worst, given what they were touching, with outright lechery.[30] In these texts, a practitioner's touch gets reconceptualized to become newly aligned with the masculine attributes of reason and decorous action; the generating woman gets repositioned as the generally silent, material object of a practitioner's magisterial ministrations; and a refashioned image of the midwife emerges—as someone who is self-sufficient, possessed of native authority, and powerfully effective in the world of action by a unique ability to subjugate body to mind, practice to knowledge.

■ Percival Willughby was a practicing physician and male midwife in both London and Derby in the mid-to-late seventeenth century. Toward the end of his career and over a period of about a decade, he wrote up what was later published as his *Observations in Midwifery*, which offers practical advice in the art of midwifery based on and demonstrated by 150 case histories.[31] The text as a whole makes two basic points: first, in normal deliveries, midwives are not to interfere in the process of birth, that they are "but nature's servants in all their performances, and that they must attend her time and motion" (*OM*, 5). Second, when difficulty does arise, either because of obstruction or malpresentation, midwives should perform what Willughby calls "the handy operation"(*OM*, 1), or podalic version, a method of manually turning an infant to a foot presentation, which allows a practitioner to grab hold of a leg and effect delivery by exerting traction.

Throughout the text, Willughby seeks to distinguish himself from the general cast of midwives by relying on the superior status of intellectual over manual labor and by evoking the mutually exclusive associations of each. Willughby, who works with his head, is rational and effective, a man most nearly associated with mind; midwives, who work with their hands, are dangerously intrusive and aggressive. Touch, a capacity of the body, is thus marked as both female and vulgar. Yet Willughby himself advocates "the handy operation," and he wants midwives to learn it as well. So he must somehow endorse *his* engagement in the body and in manual labor, and still distinguish it from the normative labor of midwives. Over the course of the 150 cases he describes, Willughby accomplishes this paradoxical conceptual design by performing two contradictory rhetorical maneuvers. He contrasts himself to other midwives first by setting his compassionate *rational* labor against their aggressive *manual* labor, but then he ascribes to *his* manual labor the attributes of reason; he too works with his hands, but his hands, unlike those of meddlesome midwives, are ever guided by his head. The result is a man identified with reason and mind but able to *use* rather than be delimited by his body.

Willughby claims he has learned from experience that in most cases, midwives do best when they do least, forbearing from any interference in a delivery. That midwives have not themselves sufficiently learned this lesson he demonstrates in his characterization of their intrusive handiwork. Early on in his treatise, for example, he recounts the story of Dorothy North, who, "being great with child, was afflicted with some disquiets in her belly":

> Severall midwives were called to assist her; one of them thrust up her hand, and made great struggling in her body; at the taking of it forth, her hand was all over bloody, and this midwife made great vaunts of her skil, and doings, and said, That the Child did stick to the woman's back, but that shee had removed it.
>
> At my coming, I found that the waters had not flowed, and that the womb was closed; I gave her a milky clyster that much abated her paines. I instructed one of the milder sort, that was left alone with her, what to do, and what to observe, and intreated her to bee gentle and patient with the woman, and to stay the appointed time, assuring her, That the fruit would fall off it-self, when that it was full ripe.

Some two or three dayes after my departure, shee was well delivered by this
midwife, but her child was dead. (*OM*, 7)

The midwife who precedes him at the labor acts with both unthinking aggression and unjust self-promotion: she "thrust up her hand," "struggl[ed]" within
the woman's body, removed her hand "all over bloody," yet nonetheless "made
great vaunts of her skil." Willughby by contrast uses his head; all the verbs that
describe his actions indicate the considered rationality of his behavior. Where
the midwife thrust and made vaunts, Willughby "found," "instructed," and
"intreated" the midwife "to be gentle and patient." And though he presumably
did perform a manual examination to determine that "the womb was closed,"
he entirely occludes this bodily contact from the case. The rhetorical effect of
the absence of Willughby's hand underscores the contrast he constructs between
himself and the midwife already present. She, who thrusts her hand, is associated with violence, haste, and self-promotion; he, who seemingly uses only his
head, is associated with compassion, patience, and modesty.

Having thus affiliated his efforts with the rational intellect, Willughby must
shift his self-presentation when he comes explicitly to recount his own manual
interventions in delivery. In contrast to the typical midwife who, having quickly
"daubed" her hands with oil, is given to "haling . . . pulling, and stretching"
women's bodies, Willughby seems quite the gentleman, instructing midwives
instead to "slide" their hands "anointed with oil" into a woman's womb (*OM*,
6). In recounting his delivery of a woman who had been in labor for three days
before his arrival, Willughby describes how

. . . between the child's head, and her body, I put my two fingers, and lifted up the
skin toward the fundament over the child's head. Then it pleased God to suffer the
child's head to slide into the world. (*OM*, 61)

Compared to the midwives who stretch the parts and thrust up their hands,
Willughby's manual maneuvers seem as gentle as they are efficient. His actions
are both deliberate and moderated, and, presumably because of this, his manual intervention becomes the medium for achieving God's ends: lifting up the
skin as if it were a veil, Willughby reveals the child beneath and thus makes it
possible for God to permit its birth. Willughby's instructions on how to perform
"the handy operation" similarly attempt to refashion the hand's associations with
unthinking aggression. A midwife is told, in reducing an arm presentation, "lea-

surely to slide up her anointed hand over the child's arme, and gently to force it upward" (*OM*, 92); elsewhere, he advises that if "you have a desire to turn the child, when that it hath too great a head," you should

> Slide up your hand anointed into the woman's body, and, afterward, spread it flat upon the child's head, and gently force the child back . . . until you have roome enough to search for the feet, and having found a foot, draw it leasurely forth, holding the foot in your hand griped [sic] between your fingers. The infant's body will turn easily round, and so bee drawn forth. (*OM*, 75)

Willughby's recourse here and elsewhere to the oxymoron "to gently force" suggests the rhetorical struggle he is engaged in, to make the obstetrical hand an instrument of gentility and leisure. In striving to do so, Willughby strives as well to make of himself an expert practitioner whose manual skills are not opposed to but are rather the subservient vehicles of a reasoned and deliberate mind.

The hand, for Willughby, was primarily a mechanical tool, a means of making possible the delivery of live births in difficult labors. When Henrik van Deventer's 1701 treatise on midwifery was published in English in 1716, the hand became an epistemological tool as well. Deventer's innovation was to use internal examination, what he called "the Touch," to determine not only the position of the fetus in the womb, but also the orientation of the womb in the pelvis.[32] Deventer emphasized the importance of knowing both general pelvic anatomy and the particular characteristics of an individual woman's pelvic structure.[33] Along with this knowledge he also advocated the technique of manually manipulating the mother's coccyx, which would slightly enlarge the birth canal and thus ease the delivery.[34]

Although he recognized that his knowledge of how to "handle a woman in labor" (*AMI*, 215) was not without flaws, it transgressed the norms of modesty (*AMI*, 250), for example, and occasionally yielded incorrect information (*AMI*, 156), Deventer insists that the touch is the best means of knowing the status of a woman's labor and of whether any difficulty will arise.

Unlike many of the midwifery texts of the period, which seem to assume that learning to know by touch would be accomplished through experience, Deventer offers fairly detailed and specific instructions on how to perform "the Touch." He says, for example, that you can know "whether the womb and the infant are directly or ill situated for Birth" by performing the following procedure:

Their Fingers being plentifully and smoothly besmeared, are to be passed through the Lips of the Privities gently separated, into the Vagina, taking Care, lest they force their Fingers or Nails against the Sides or other Parts, giving way as much as they can to the Wrinkles, or any other things which lie in the way, following the strait Passage, tending downwards rather than upwards, against the Neck of the Bladder, till the Fingers slipping gently and gradually betwixt the Neck of the Bladder and the strait Gut, touch the Mouth or bottom of the Womb which resists them, whose Form they may exactly feel and measure with the ends of their Fingers. (*AMI*, 79–80)[35]

By following these fairly precise instructions, a midwife can determine whether the head or some other part will emerge first and thus know, in advance, whether the delivery will be easy or difficult. The advantage of touch, in other words, is that it provides certainty where none would be otherwise possible. The "eminent physician" who wrote the preface to Deventer's treatise indicates as much in his praise for the work. Deventer's "directions about Touching Women before they Labour," he says, makes this a guide "whereby [midwives] may foresee all Difficulties as they happen, and prevent them early from becoming greater by an otherwise unavoidable Surprize" (*AMI*, A5r). Touching provides the ability to see the future, to foresee "all" difficulty. The one who touches is thereby in the unique position of knowing what the others assembled in the birthing room do not; the hand affords the privilege of knowledge.

It is possible to see the rhetorical effects of this epistemological advantage in Deventer's description of "How it may be known by the Touch, whether a Woman be with Child or not" (*AMI*, 65). The problem a practitioner faced, as we saw in chapter 5, was that the conventional signs of impregnation were not altogether certain. As Deventer says, "though the stopping of the Courses, vomiting, loss of Appetite, a depraved Appetite, the swelling of the Breasts, pain of the Nipples, and at last, the swelling of the Belly are looked upon as the surest and most known Signs, yet very often we find them common with those that are not with Child, and Virgins, as well as Women with Child" (*AMI*, 65). These signs, available either to the woman herself (cessation of the menses, loss of appetite, pain in the breasts) or to everyone who sees her (swelling of the breasts and belly), are not to be relied upon. Instead, says Deventer,

The most certain Signs of Impregnation, especially in the last Months, are to be supplied by the Touch; therefore a Woman, who is uncertain of her Conception, and is desirous to know whether she hath conceived or not, whether any of the above-mentioned Signs appear or not . . . it is to be tried by the Touch, that you may truly know, whether the Matter be so. (*AMI*, 66)

After stating the basic proposition—that touch supplies the certain signs—Deventer attends to a woman's desire: "therefore a woman, who is . . . desirous to know. . . . " But when touch is tried, it provides certainty not to the woman, but to "you," the midwife who touches. Touch, in other words, becomes the medium through which the woman's desire fades into the practitioner's intellectual dominance. And what was once a form of communal knowledge, the traditional but uncertain signs of conception, becomes the exclusive knowledge of the practitioner.

The increasingly exclusive prominence of the midwife in relation to the childbearing woman and other practitioners present in the birthing room is apparent also in Deventer's instructions for how to perform basic diagnoses about labor. Like Willughby, Deventer believed that in natural births a midwife performs her function if she only "receives the Infant, cuts off the Navel-string, takes care of the Infant by washing and nourishing it, or recommends that to be done by any of the Gossips" (*AMI*, 91). But, unlike Willughby, who not infrequently determines the status of a labor by *talking* both to the midwives already present and to the childbearing woman herself, Deventer knows whatever is necessary by touch alone. He thus teaches that the first thing a midwife is to do upon entering the birthing room is determine the woman's physical state by performing a manual examination:

> As soon as [a midwife] comes to a woman in labour, in the beginning, I say, her duty will be, first, to try the woman by the touch, by which means she may presently judge accurately of the situation of the womb and infant, viz. whether one is well turned, and the other well placed; and to find out by sense, whether the pelvis be large or small, round or plain, and how the womb is placed, and the infant turned upon it, or in it; in which cases they are to do all they can, that without delay, if occasion requires it, the Infant may be drawn out artificially by hand; or the exclusion is to be waited for by the pains alone, or nature is to be assisted; art supplying what she is wanting in. (*AMI*, 124)

The description is of an entirely silent encounter between the parts of a woman's body (her womb and pelvis), the infant, and a midwife who makes a diagnosis "by sense." If traditionally the testimony of the childbearing woman herself was necessary to a complete assessment of any birth ceremony, now all that needs to be known is determined by touch.

This is not to say that the mother's participation in the birth process is occluded altogether in Deventer's text. Deventer believed that birth is the result of the combined efforts of the infant's desire to be released (*AMI*, 155), the womb's contractions (what he calls "effectual pain"), and, in difficult cases, the midwife's "artificial hand." But the efforts of the others engaged in the process of childbirth are routinely subordinated to the practitioner's art. For example, in describing his technique in obstructed head presentations, Deventer portrays both the mother and the midwife as together enacting the birth, but success seems assured only in the midwife's hands. After describing the "middle" posture, "betwixt sitting and lying down" in which he places the woman, Deventer depicts his technique of manipulating the mother's coccyx and its happy results:

> then I thrust up my whole hand, first put into oil, or well anointed with it. . . . My hands being put up, I turn the palm upwards, and the back of it downwards towards the Intestinum Rectum or strait gut, and the Os Sacrum: by this means, I put my fingers as far as I can to the head, rather thrusting it a little backwards, than it should hinder me from placing my hand well and firmly against the Os Coccygis. My hand being so placed, I advise the woman not to let her pains pass to no purpose, but endeavour with all her power: as soon then as I perceive the pain coming on (which I commonly perceive before the woman) then I thus advise her, *now the pains are just coming on, make use of them, press down with all your force, I will help you*: When I have said this, I gradually press my Hand backwards, and now and then more strongly against the point of the Os Sacrum, bring it downwards at the same time, that may give way to the head as it slides down; and the more violent the pains, the more I press down; and the more I press down with effectual pain, the more strongly the woman is able to labour. By this means, and the womans violent pressing downwards, and by enlarging the passage, and by bringing my hand back, the infant's head sliding down succeeds and follows it; this I repeat as often as the case requires it, no pain being spent in vain; by this means the woman, who already finds help, takes courage, especially if upon every pain, I tell her, *Things go well and prosper in my hands, we shall presently congratulate you a joyful mother*. The woman in labour being thus encouraged, who just before had cast away all Hopes, is now so much strengthened, that collecting all her might, she does her best endeavours; by which means the infant is soon brought forth. (*AMI*, 134–35)

Clearly, the childbearing woman participates actively in this account of delivery, and Deventer clearly recognizes her as an agent in the process, needing her to "make use" of her pains and verbally encouraging her to press downwards. But it is also clear that the woman is in the "hands" of the midwife, both figuratively and literally. With his hands, the midwife establishes the status of the womb, the position of the infant, the structure of the pelvis, and whether or not the "artificial hand" that manipulates the mother's body will be necessary. "Things go well and prosper in my hands," he says, confident of the future (he knows in advance of the mother when her pains are coming on) and suggesting obliquely a sense of salvation. She had "cast away all Hopes," but is now assured of imminent "joy." Wholly in control of the birthing process, Deventer is the unquestioned authority in the encounter, a man of knowledge and compassion, a man of dexterity offering deliverance.

Willughby and Deventer advocate manual techniques to replace the need for the destructive instruments of obstetrical surgeons, who were called upon to extract presumably dead infants with hooks and crochets. In their different ways—Willughby by urging the use of podalic version (the handy operation) and Deventer by urging manual examination and manipulation of the mother's body (the touch)—both male midwives seek to deliver living children in birthing situations that might otherwise result in the death of the infant, the mother, or both. The identities they construct are based precisely on the power they assign to the combined effects of an established subjugation: hand to head, experience to intellect. Even their admissions of failure add to their constructed subjectivities; these are reasonable men, men enough to admit their mistakes.

Willughby and Deventer were physicians as well as a male midwives, so, theoretically at least, their aim in writing their texts was not so much to replace the office of the midwife as to change some of its standard techniques. In the 1730s, however, two books on midwifery were published that were more explicitly intended to delimit the midwife's role. Edmund Chapman and William Giffard were the first two to announce in print the uses of the forceps, an instrument that had been secretly used by the Chamberlen family for several generations and was reputed to be able to aid in the delivery of obstructed head presentations. As obstetrical surgeons, their practice would have been generally limited to emergency situations, when the life of the parturient woman was thought to be in imminent danger. But the forceps made it at least theoretically possible for an obstetrical surgeon to deliver an obstructed infant alive, if, among other things, the surgeon was called in early enough to save it. Thus, although both men claim to be writing to educate midwives, they seem to want most to urge midwives, as Chapman says, to "send early for Advice upon the Appearance of Danger and Difficulty" (*IM*, preface). Seeking therefore to restrict the role of midwives to normal deliveries and to expand the role of surgeons, both authors seek an exclusive authority, an autonomy established against a diminished or degraded female presence.

Chapman announces at the beginning of his text, *Essay on the Improvement of Midwifery*, that midwives should make themselves masters of the forceps or the fillet, a related instrument of his own invention. Such knowledge is crucial, he claims, because when difficult births cannot be effected by the hand alone, they can be accomplished with the aid of these instruments, which, he says, are perfectly safe and innocent (*IM*, preface). Yet rather than teaching midwives how to use the instruments or perform manual version, Chapman trains his attention on his own exquisite achievements in childbirth. Although, like Willughby, he occasionally admits committing some mistakes (as when he accidentally "snapped" a child's arm in an effort to extract it) (*IM*, 58), he generally comes off less as a conscientious practitioner advocating a particular point of view about medical practice than as the self-proclaimed hero of a series of medical dramas.

Chapman's astonishing talents are most obviously manifest in his repeated assertions of the "great ease" with which he routinely effects difficult deliveries. When a woman is unable to deliver after several hours of effort, Chapman determines that it is

> necessary to have recourse to Art, and so with great ease as well to my patient as to my self, [I] passed my hand, and in one minute delivered her of the child. (*IM*, 55)

Entirely avoiding any information about what precisely he did when he "passed [his] hand" into the woman's body, Chapman's focus is on his own accomplishment—a one-minute delivery of a child the woman could not herself produce after hours of exertion. In another case, Chapman describes the history of a woman who had two or three times been delivered of obstructed head presentations by a man who used the hook to extract them. At her next labor, Chapman was called in early; finding that although the child lay in the right posture, it "made no advance," Chapman receives permission to use art:

> I now had leave to act as I should think fit; upon which I put the woman in a proper posture . . . then gently passing my hand into the womb, I took the child by the feet, and so delivered her in two or three minutes, with great ease and safety. (*IM*, 54)

This time we hear in general terms what he does with his hand in the woman's womb; he takes the child by the feet. But how does he do this? How does he find the feet? How does he turn the child in the womb? The lack of instructional detail only highlights Chapman's unparalleled accomplishment: his delivery "with great ease" in "two or three minutes" of a woman who previously had to suffer the surgeon's hook.

Chapman's touch, it would seem, is being stylized in these cases as a mechanism for medical efficiency. A practitioner passes his hand into a woman's womb, but we, as readers, are made to imagine not the actual, material mess of that touch—the waters and blood of birth—but rather the remarkable efficacy of a medical man's prowess. In the process of being purified of its associations with manual labor, with matter, with the body itself, the practitioner's touch bequeaths a power that is meant to mark incontestable efficiency and authority precisely because it is so purified; paradoxically, the body is enlisted precisely in order to be superceded.

The authority that Chapman's touch confers is, appropriately, more aligned with rational justice than with any sense of physical coercion, given that it is built from but also independent of the body. That this is so is evident from his descriptions of what ensues when his authority is not followed. In the case of a clergyman's wife, for example, who "had a sudden discharge of some ounces of blood from the womb" in the seventh month of her pregnancy, Chapman's warnings "both to her and her Husband" that she was in mortal danger went unheeded. He was therefore not permitted "to have the liberty to do as [he] judged proper," which was to extract the infant "by art." By the time he was called back to the woman's house, therefore, it was "too late": the woman was seized with violent flooding, and, though he was able to deliver her "in less than one minute," the "unhappy wilful Lady was lost . . . " (IM, 59–61). The woman dies, in other words, because of what Chapman presents as the obvious stupidity of the balance of power in the birthing room. Clearly, he knows both first and best; he knows that a detached placenta is causing her "flooding" and that it threatens her life. But though he implies that his superior knowledge should grant him authority, he must attend upon the wishes of the family; they must grant him the "liberty to do as [he] judge[s] proper." The suggestion is that it is both unjust and dangerous to subject Chapman's inherent "liberty" and earned authority to the uninformed wishes of others, not least those of a "wilful Lady."

The fact that Chapman narrates his cases in a way that consistently maximizes the legitimacy of his implicit claim to authority and intellectual mastery does not mean that he occludes entirely the experience of the expectant mother. Indeed, the sufferings of the mother are everywhere apparent in Chapman's record, from the "poor tender-hearted mother" forced to see her child "brought in the world a cripple" when a male midwife "lopped off" its presenting arm because he mistakenly believed the child to be dead, to the "young healthy mother cut off in the bloom of life and cast into the cold arms of death, just as she was about to clasp her first-born in her own" because the midwife tore out her "matrix" having mistaken it for an afterbirth "stuck" inside her (*IM*, 31, 83–84). But his recourse to melodrama ("tender-hearted mother," "bloom of life," "cold arms of death") only underscores his own heroics; tales of woeful mothers are depicted to advance his polemic against competing practitioners, both men and women, surgeons and midwives, who, it seems, needlessly torture women already in distress. Thus his sympathetic portrayal of childbearing women works to advance his own self-construction as an obstetrical hero—he comes, with hand and tool, equipped with the unique ability to relieve "in a minute or two" the dire sufferings of women.

If Chapman constructs the mother as a hapless victim in order to advance the lessons of his own heroics, William Giffard takes another tack to achieve quite similar results, nearly effacing the mother altogether or reducing her to a litany of body parts. Although most of the 225 cases he recounts in his posthumously published *Cases in Midwifery* do not involve the use of what are called "Mr. Giffard's extractors" (plate 12, page 181), the first case in which he describes using them successfully neatly demonstrates the rhetorical relation between the practitioner's touch and the mother's absence:

June the 28th, 1728. I was called upon to go to see a poor Woman in Labour: the Midwife told me the Pains were short, with long intervals. I felt her pulse, which was regular and strong, and upon Touching her, found the Child to present its Head, but high: . . . the next morning I . . . found the Child but little advanced, her pulse very quick and labouring, and the Womb very much spread, so that I could entirely pass my Fingers round the Head to the Ears, for it was no ways engaged, but loose; the Vagina was large, she having had seven or eight Children before; wherefore considering that her pulse grew languid, and that her strength decreased, I thought it advisable to attempt her Delivery. I endeavoured to press the child back, that I might be able to turn it and get the Feet; but it was so locked at the shoulders, I was not able to move it; whereupon I passed my Extractor and drew it with much difficulty forwards without the Labia, and then taking hold of the Head on each side with my

Hands (which cannot be done whilst it lies in the Vagina) I drew the shoulders out; the other parts readily followed. . . . The Child was born alive.[36]

In the scene Giffard conjures up, the childbearing woman is simply a "poor Woman in Labour" who, after her initial introduction, fades from the case as a coherent entity. Other than conferring with the midwife, Giffard's interactions are entirely with body parts rather than with a person. The mother's absence from the story even registers grammatically: after saying that "the midwife told [him] that the pains were short," Giffard says, "I felt her pulse . . . and upon Touching her, found the Child to present its Head." Although the context demands that the repeated "her" refer to the woman in labor, she has been excised from the rhetorical reconstruction of the scene; therefore, the grammatical antecedent of the pronouns is, illogically, the midwife. This grammatical glitch recurs in the next sentence as well, in which the only and absurd antecedent of the "her" in "her pulse" is the Child. By the time we hear something of the woman's history, that she has had seven or eight children before, she seems an attenuated extrapolation of body parts and functions: vagina large, womb spread, pulse strong or languid. The woman simply does not exist in the case history as a complete, coherent person; Giffard never speaks to her, gleaning nearly all his information by touching her parts, and, unlike the child whose fate we learn, the woman's outcome is unrevealed. Although it is not always the case that the childbearing woman is entirely absent from Giffard's text—we might learn, for example, that a woman died from flooding because midwives did not know to call him early enough or that a woman "recovered very fast" after he revived her with "the use of proper Cordials"—she is rarely presented as volitional (*CM*, 62, 72). Agency is transferred to Giffard, whose cases record his efforts with wombs, infants, and extractors, but not per se with mothers.

I am trying to point to a pattern in the midwifery case histories of the late seventeenth and early eighteenth centuries in which the construction of a practitioner's authority emerges as the effect of a new reliance on touch and a newly imagined network of associations for touch. In the common rhetorical maneuvers of these texts, touch creates an image of the medical practitioner that contrasts sharply with what we know about the practice of medicine at the time. Whereas medicine generally and childbirth in particular were essentially communal endeavors, these case histories typically construct an individualized and exclusive expertise for their authors. The claim to this authority is based on the superior knowledge that touch generates, which allows the practitioner to offer

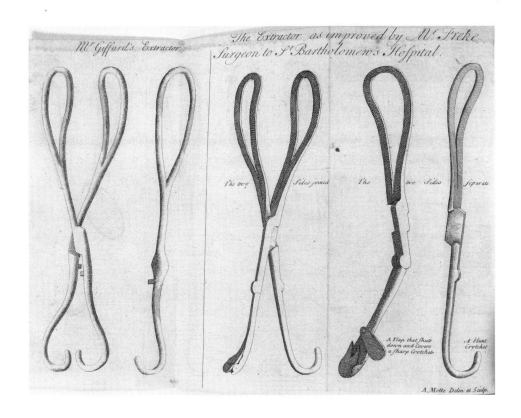

*Plate 12. From William Giffard's* Cases in Midwifery *(London, 1734), the plate depicts Mr.*

*Giffard's extractors. Reproduced by permission of the New York Academy of Medicine Library.*

diagnoses that the others collected in the birthing room generally either do not know, deny, or cannot even fathom. The effect is moreover compounded by the rhetorical manipulation of arguably the most important subject in the birthing room, namely the childbearing woman, who is conceived either as a victim in need of heroic rescue or, more dramatically, as an array of body parts confidently prodded by the practitioner.

Considered collectively, the medical practitioners that emerge from these rhetorical patterns form a fairly familiar identity, one possessed of individual sovereignty, rational prowess, and discrete manual dexterity, who can handle, with patience and efficiency, crucial moments in life and death. This, paradigmatically, is the early modern, even the Enlightenment hero, who, having sought knowledge from books, values equally the knowledge of experience, who is endowed with a native liberty that only the ignorant would deny, and who, because of that knowledge and the exercise of that liberty, is able to be generous and compassionate toward those who suffer. This is of course a masculine model more than a generically human one, and the construction of this model in the texts of male practitioners who were making their way into a workplace that had previously been exclusively female suggests the importance of gender in the process of its construction. But the gender issue here is not simply tied to the sex of the competing practitioners, because the rhetorical effect of this model is to generate *medical* authority even as it evokes a mode of masculine identity. I am arguing, in other words, that medical authority gets established in the birthing room as the agents who practice there represent themselves, regardless of their sex, in accordance with emerging ideals of masculine subjectivity. And I am arguing further that the subtle rhetorical manipulations of the new techniques of touch, precisely because they collectively permit the association of the practitioner with a hierarchical alignment of *both* mental and manual power, are instrumental in the generation of this unprecedented authority.

That a disembodied touch is a key mechanism for creating a medical authority attuned to masculine identity is nicely demonstrated in the work of Sarah Stone, whose collection of forty case histories, published in 1737, contains what is perhaps the most exaggerated version of this construction. Keenly aware of the gender politics of her profession, Stone addresses her treatise to her "sisters," warning against the embarrassment and danger of exposing oneself to the "boyish Pretenders" in the field, who, at best, derive their knowledge of women's bodies by "dissecting the Dead" and necessarily lack the "natural Sympathy" that exists among women who "have gone thro the Pangs of Childbearing" (*CPM*, vii, xiv–xv). Stone considers men inadequate for the job of midwifery and believes that, with the proper education, female midwives will be able to "deliver in difficult labours, as well as those that are not so," which in turn will keep women from being "forced to send for a Man"(*CPM*, ix, vi). The elaborate title of her book gives a sense of what she thinks of its contents:

A complete practice of midwifery, [which includes, in addition to] forty cases . . . selected from many others, in the course of a very extensive practice, many necessary cautions and useful instructions, proper to be observed in the most dangerous and critical exigencies, as well when the delivery is difficult in its own nature, as when it becomes so by the rashness or ignorance of unexperienc'd pretenders.

Stone intends her book to provide precisely the education midwives need to keep them from being forced to call on men, and her forty cases serve as exempla: this is what I did in this difficult instance; do the same and you will not need men. But rather than provide the advertised education, the text works hardest to create an authoritative image of Stone herself.

Her very first "observation" sets the pattern:

At Bridgewater, Somersetshire, 1703. I was sent for the Huntspill, to a Farmer's wife, who had been in Labour three days: her pains were declining, and she reduced to the utmost degree of weakness; not having been in Bed all that time, (which is the common, but very bad, practice of the country midwives.) When I came, I found her spirits quite exhausted; and her midwife, being also fatigued, was in a sound sleep. I laid the Woman on the Bed, and by Touching her, found the Child lay on the Os Pubis (or share-bone). The Waters being gone, made the remaining part of her Labour the more difficult: however, relieving her Child from the Os Pubis, which strengthen'd her pains, I deliver'd her of a Daughter alive, and that in the space of three hours; to the grand surprise of her Midwife, when awake, who seem'd glad the Child was born alive, she believing it dead the day before. (*CPM*, 1–2)

We have here all the by-now familiar elements: a woman exhausted and in danger, and a typically incompetent country midwife who sleeps through her patient's decline. In the context of this exhaustion—the others have, it seems, given up, and the midwife believes the child to be dead—Stone is all action and determination; she is the subject of all the active verbs in the story: I came, I found, I laid, I deliver'd. Stone's success is due to her "Touching," since it is that touch that shows her that the child lies on the share-bone, but she provides no information at all either on how to touch to determine the child's position or on how to remove the child from the share-bone. So what lesson is taught here? What about midwifery is a reader to learn from this "observation"? When others sleep, Stone moves to action.

Again, Stone is called to a shoemaker's wife. She finds her in so "deplorable" a condition that all her friends have given her over to death. Says Stone: "I touch'd her, and assur'd them all, that, with God's assistance, I did not doubt of delivering her in two hours; which I accordingly did: both Mother and Child did well" (*CPM*, 12). Here Stone seems nearly divine; merely by touching the woman, she somehow knows the future (that she will deliver the woman in two hours) and performs an apparent miracle: the delivery of child from mother and mother from death. Without any information about how or where to touch a laboring woman, Stone's educative project is belied; her rhetorical use of touch is purely in the service of her own self-construction. Only she touches, only she knows, only she does, so only she succeeds. Effacing the material detail of the bodies themselves, touch in these cases seems less like a specific manual maneuver than like a disembodied mode of medical magic, and the practitioner who performs that magic seems not simply the rational hero of a medical enlightenment, but more nearly the wonder-working hero of medical myth. Though a woman, Stone fashions herself in the image of modern man.

After the 1730s, men increasingly entered the profession of midwifery, but their rise to medical prominence was neither easy nor swift. The resistance came from female midwives, who derided their reliance on instruments and denounced them as patent dangers, but also and increasingly from men who, deeply suspicious of the art of touching, condemned male midwifery as an only barely disguised indulgence in sexual license.[37] That male-midwifery gradually overcame these obstacles, evolving eventually into the field of obstetrics, was due to a combination of social forces. Especially in well-to-do areas of cities like London, male midwives were thought to be superior to their female counterparts both because of their access to formal education and because of their advertised skills in using costly instruments that enabled them to handle successfully difficult as well as normal deliveries. But these early collections of case histories add another aspect to this already gendered story. Read rhetorically, they epitomize the relation between generating bodies and gendered selves in early modern England: touching the body of a childbearing woman, the practitioner is newly made, a self-determining, rational individual. And the generative female, always aligned in the bio-medical literature of the time with the womb, with the "mother," becomes the mother of modern man, rhetorically fashioned as the fount from which the masculine subject of western modernity is born.

# EPILOGUE

N LATE JANUARY, 2005, SENATOR SAM BROWNBACK (R-Kansas), along with over thirty cosponsors, introduced into the United States Senate a bill called the "Unborn Child Pain Awareness Act of 2005" (S.51).[1] Based on "findings" that "unborn children" of twenty-weeks gestation or more are "pain-capable," the bill, if passed, will require abortion providers to ensure that pregnant women whose fetuses are past twenty weeks gestation be informed of the following:

> that "the Congress of the United States has determined" that an "unborn child" at this stage of development can "experience pain";

> that Congress finds that there is "substantial evidence" that the process of "being killed in an abortion will cause the unborn child pain"; and

> that you [the woman seeking an abortion] have the "option of choosing to have anesthesia or other pain-reducing drug or drugs administered directly to the pain-capable unborn child. . . ."

This "information" will be delivered to the pregnant woman both verbally and in a pamphlet prepared by the Department of Health and Human Services. If the woman decides to continue with the abortion, she will further have to sign an "Unborn Child Pain Awareness Decision Form," which the provider will be required to keep on file. The form will indicate the woman's explicit request for or denial of anesthesia for her "pain-capable unborn child." Penalties for noncompliance range between $100,000 (for a first violation) to $250,000 (for subsequent violations), along with suspension or revocation of one's medical license.

"Pro-life" advocates have been forthright about their intentions in crafting and promoting this bill. Spurred by the signing into law of the Partial Birth Abortion Ban in 2003, supporters of the Unborn Child Pain Awareness Act see this bill as the next step in what they claim to be an evolving expression among Americans of the "unconditional love" that pervades "the greatest human rights movement on Earth."[2]

The bill's prospects are uncertain. Its logic is questionable: it projects as medical facts issues that are the subject of debate in the medical community. Moreover, it conscripts abortion providers to deliver biased, government mandated speeches. Congress thus has many reasons to reject it. But Congress has not been ruled by reason on this issue, as is demonstrated by its repeated passage of the Partial Birth Abortion Ban, only to watch it succumb to federal court challenges. If congress passes the Unborn Child Pain Awareness Act, its fate will eventually also be determined in the federal courts, which are themselves in flux on the question of constitutional protection for abortion rights. Whatever its chances of being enforced as law, however, the bill remains provocative, not least because of the language of its presentation.

In the section on Definitions, the bill defines an "unborn child" as "a member of the species homo sapiens, *at any stage of development*, who is carried in the womb" (Sec. 2901; emphasis mine). Though the bill covers only fetuses at or over twenty weeks, the definition of what comprises a "child" covers "any stage of development." The implicit claim here is not simply that "life" begins at conception, but that childhood does. Like Kerckring over three hundred years ago, this bill grants not just life, but *childhood* to an embryo. What was new in the seventeenth century—the endowment of embryos with attributes of personhood—has become a given in the language of a piece of twenty-first century legislation.

And here is the definition of "woman": "a female human being who is capable of becoming pregnant, whether or not she has reached the age of majority." According to this formulation, a post-menopausal female, a female who has undergone hysterectomy or become infertile following chemotherapy is not a woman, but a ten-year-old who has reached menarche is. Here the implicit logic of the early modern bio-medical woman reaches what is perhaps its fullest elaboration; it is not simply a womb that defines a woman in this bill, but specifically a fertile womb. A female who cannot reproduce is simply not a woman.

■ This book has focused on a fairly localized topic—the emergence of modern notions of gendered subjectivity in and through the vernacular bio-medical literature of early modern England. But its underlying assumption, that body- and self-constructs are mutually dependent, that each always enables and entails the other, has a rather more general applicability. At the start of the book, I sought to suggest the truth of this truism by touching briefly on new (or, I would want to say, renewed) notions of body and self evident in certain versions of the posthuman. And embodied, networked selves are in fact now presiding in numerous academic arena, not just in humanities departments but also, and especially, in computer labs, in neuroscience centers, even in departments of architecture. As William Mitchell, a theorist of the networked city, has neatly put it, "I link, therefore I am."[3]

But even here, even in a sophistocated discussion of the cyborg self in a networked urban environment, one can still hear traces of the early modern model that Senator Brownback makes so explicit in his recent bill. Demonstrating the hyperconnectivity of our increasingly networked cities, Mitchell describes himself as follows:

> I am inextricably entangled in the networks of my air, water, waste disposal, energy, transportation, and Internet service providers.[4]

Some pages later he elaborates:

> Through electronic storage and distribution of my encoded commands—particularly by means of digital networks—I can indefinitely multiply and distribute my points of physical agency through space and time.[5]

Both sentences demonstrate the embeddedness of the "I" in the physical and information webs of contemporary networked culture. And, though he takes himself as his example, Mitchell's "I" is theoretically ungendered. But both sentences also conceptually separate the "I" from the network. "I" am "entangled in networks"; "I" extend "my . . . agency" through space and time. This is not the constitution of the self in and through the network, but the extended efficiency and power of the "I" by means of the network. This is an updated, twenty-first century version of a historically masculine supervenience: the "I" that precedes and commands a network. "I link, therefore I am" permutes but does not ultimately undo the *cogito*.

True, this is a style of speaking, as is the definitional terminology of Senator Brownback's proposed legislation. Mitchell does thoroughly argue for the cyborg self—a self constituted by its connectivity. And I suspect that Senator Brownback, if pressed, would admit that the category "woman" does in fact include infertile females. But my methodological assumption, at its most basic level, has been simply that words matter, that words actually reveal something of what and how we think. And if that truism also is true, then the words of Senator Brownback and William Mitchell, though surely spoken from the otherwise disparate perspectives of the humanist and the posthuman condition, nonetheless together disclose the tenacity of the early modern; they tell us how deeply entrenched we are in the models of gendered selfhood whose generation in the rhetoric of early modern bio-medicine I have in this book sought to describe.

Summer, 2006

# NOTES

## Introduction

1 Throughout this book, I use the term
*bio-medical* to refer both to biological
theory and research and to medical
practice. I use a hyphen to indicate
the difference between my usage of
the term and its more common and
restricted meaning as the application
of the natural sciences to clinical medicine. "Bio-medical writing" thus refers
to a diverse body of texts that together
treat the theoretical and the practical
aspects of what in the early modern
period was called "physic." Early modern texts also speak of "generation"
rather than "reproduction." As I will
discuss in chapter 5, the latter term
became current only after the physiological processes from conception
through birth came to be understood
within the context of mechanism. By
*vernacular* texts I specifically mean texts
in English, whether they were initially
written in English or were translations
of texts originally written in another
language. Social historians frequently
use the term to indicate an opposition
to *learned* texts, with a meaning closer
to *popular*, so that vernacular texts are
those written for a wide and frequently
lay reading public. Some of the texts I
will consider here fit that sense of the
vernacular (for example, the midwifery
manuals I consider in chapter 3), but
many do not. Helkiah Crooke (chapter
2) said he was writing specifically for
surgeons; Harvey (chapter 4) wrote his
book on the generation of animals in
Latin for the learned medical establishment in both England and Europe,
though his book was translated into
English soon after it was published;
*Philosophical Transactions of the Royal
Society* (chapter 5) was mostly published
in English but included translations
from Latin and from European vernac-
ulars. The genres I engage here are
diverse; the audiences implied in the
texts only sometimes overlap. I write
about vernacular—English language—
texts because these permit a rhetorical
analysis that, I hope to show, points to
widespread cultural patterns that per-
sist across generic divides.

2 The scholarship on early modern subjectivity is vast, stretching back at least
as far as the nineteenth century to
Jacob Burckhardt's *The Civilization of
the Renaissance in Italy* (1859; repr.,
Oxford: Phaidon, 1981). For Burckhardt,
the Renaissance saw the birth of the
individual, a coherent and authentic
self released from the constraints of
religion and custom, newly freed to
find its expression and realization out-

side a primary identification with community. Though it still has its supporters (for example, Robin Kirkpatrick, in *The European Renaissance, 1400–1600* [London: Longman, 2002]), Burckhardt's vision has been increasingly critiqued in the past quarter of a century on both historical and sociological grounds. More recent interpretations see the Renaissance self not as a free, rational, and self-determining individual, but rather as a construct of sociopolitical forces, a self understood in terms not of authenticity but, as Stephen Greenblatt so influentially put it, of self-fashioning (*Renaissance Self-Fashioning: More to Shakespeare* [Chicago: University of Chicago Press, 1980]). For Greenblatt, the self is "remarkably unfree, the ideological product of the relations of power in a particular society" (ibid., 257). Self-presentation (in portraiture and in theater, for example) is not evidence of unitary persons displaying themselves in public to their own best advantage but rather a fragment of cultural construction, an artifact of a self divided. This model, too, has been critiqued. If Burckhardt's vision read into the Renaissance a notion of selfhood grounded in Romantic genius, Greenblatt's vision sees the Renaissance as a presaging point of the postmodern, with its delight in fragmentation and its fascination with the shifting play of surface patterns; for such a critique, see, for example, John Jeffries Martin, *Myths of Renaissance Individualism* (New York: Palgrave Macmillan, 2004). My interest here is not to determine the relative validity of either construct; I am not trying to recuperate

what the early modern subject *really* was. Rather, I want to investigate one of the discursive arenas in which the idea of the modern subject was first formulated, and I want to suggest that its formulation was integrally implicated in understandings of the gendered and generative body. In addition to the works cited above, see also C. B. MacPherson, *The Political Theory of Possessive Individualism: Hobbes to Locke* (Oxford: Clarendon Press, 1962); Charles Taylor, *Sources of the Self: The Making of Modern Identity* (Cambridge, Mass.: Harvard University Press, 1989), and Timothy Reiss, *Mirages of the Selfe: Patterns of Personhood in Ancient and Early Modern Europe* (Stanford: Stanford University Press, 2003), which I discuss later. Roy Porter, ed., *Rewriting the Self: Histories from the Renaissance to the Present* (London and New York: Routledge, 1997) is a collection of excellent essays that treats changing understandings of selfhood over a five-hundred-year period.

3  The most prolific scholars of the social history of medicine in early modern England have been Roger French, Andrew Wear, and Roy Porter. A highly selective list of important works would include the following: Roy Porter, *Patients and Practitioners: Lay Perceptions of Medicine in Pre-Industrial Society* (Cambridge: Cambridge University Press, 1985); Roy Porter and Dorothy Porter, eds., *In Sickness and in Health: The British Experience, 1650–1850* (London: The Fourth Estate, 1988); Roy Porter and Dorothy Porter, eds., *Patient's Progress: Sickness, Health and Medical Care in England, 1650–1850* (London: Polity Press, 1989); Roy Porter, ed., *The Popu-*

*larization of Medicine, 1650–1750* (London: Routledge, 1992); Andrew Wear, *Knowledge and Practice in Early Modern English Medicine, 1550–1680* (Cambridge: Cambridge University Press, 2000); Roger French, *Medicine before Science: The Rational and Learned Doctor from the Middle Ages to the Enlightenment* (Cambridge: Cambridge University Press, 2003). Harold Cook's work on the medical marketplace in seventeenth-century London remains one of the standard treatments of the subject; see *Decline of the Old Medical Regime in Stuart London* (Ithaca: Cornell University Press, 1986), 28–70. See also Margaret Pelling, *Medical Conflicts in Early Modern London: Patronage, Physicians, and Irregular Practitioners, 1550–1640* (London: Oxford University Press, 2003), which focuses on the "irregular" medical practitioners of London and their conflicts with the Royal College of Physicians. On domestic experience of sickness and household medicine, see Lucinda McCray Beier, *Sufferers and Healers: The Experience of Illness in Seventeenth-Century England* (London: Routledge & Kegan Paul, 1987) and Jennifer Stine, "Opening Closets: The Discovery of Household Medicine in Early Modern England" (PhD diss., Stanford University, 1996). On varieties of lay medical practice, see Doreen G. Nagy, *Popular Medicine in Seventeenth-Century England* (Bowling Green, Ohio: Bowling Green State University Popular Press, 1988). And on the understanding of and rituals surrounding events marking the life cycle, see David Cressy, *Birth, Marriage, and Death: Ritual, Religion, and the Life-Cycle in Tudor and Stuart England* (Oxford: Oxford Uni-

versity Press, 1997). The phrase "history from below" is Roy Porter's; see "The Patient's View: Doing Medical History from Below," *Theory and Society* 14 (1985): 175–198.

4   Mary Fissell, *Vernacular Bodies: The Politics of Reproduction in Early Modern England* (Oxford: Oxford University Press, 2004).

5   Lisa Forman Cody, *Birthing the Nation: Sex, Science, and the Conception of Eighteenth-Century Britons* (Oxford: Oxford University Press, 2005).

6   Fissell chooses to focus on cheap print texts because she wants to see popular knowledge as a "cultural artefact in its own right" (*Vernacular Bodies*, 6) rather than as a watered-down version of learned knowledge. Her study therefore demonstrates the ways in which the female reproductive body was "the material" with which ordinary people "fought battles of belief" (ibid., 41) about the religious, political, and social divisions of the time. My work, by contrast, focuses exclusively on biological and medical texts, both learned and popular, in order to trace out among many genres of medical literature a common pattern of gendered personhood. Though focused on a later period and concerned with historical events as much as with texts, Lisa Cody is interested, as I am, in the connections between questions of reproduction and the construction of identity. Cody argues against the idea that the Enlightenment public sphere was constituted by the formation of the disembodied, rational subject. By analyzing stories of the bizarre, the irrational, and especially the bodily, she proposes instead that

the body "remained vital in eighteenth century understandings of political authority, national identity, and individuals' sense of self" (*Birthing the Nation*, 7). Cody's work thus demonstrates the myth of the male subject whose formation and elaboration in the medical texts of the early modern period I explore here.

7 Thomas Laqueur, *Making Sex: Body and Gender from the Greeks to Freud* (Cambridge, Mass.: Harvard University Press, 1990). Laqueur was the first to elaborate for contemporary audiences the idea that, until the eighteenth century, the female was thought to be not an incommensurably different form but rather a homologously similar though lesser version of the male. Though his book has been much critiqued, mostly for its generalizations across time periods and specifically for its attempt to locate a shift to the two-sex model in the eighteenth century, it remains a seminal text in the history of body studies. For critiques, see Katherine Park and Robert Nye, "Destiny is Anatomy," *The New Republic* (18 February, 1991): 53–57; Meryl Altman and Keith Nightenhelser, "*Making Sex*: Review," *Postmodern Culture* 2.3 (1992); Joan Cadden, *Meanings of Sex Difference in the Middle Ages: Medicine, Science, and Culture* (Cambridge: Cambridge University Press, 1993), 2–3; Winfried Schleiner, "Early Modern Controversies about the One-Sex Model," *Renaissance Quarterly* 53 (2000): 180–91; and, most recently, Michael Stolberg, "A Woman Down to Her Bones: The Anatomy of Sexual Difference in the Sixteenth and Early Seventeenth Centuries," *Isis* 94.2 (2003): 274–99.

8 Here again the field is substantial, and I mention only a selection among the most influential studies. Gail Kern Paster, *The Body Embarrassed: Drama and the Disciplines of Shame in Early Modern Europe* (Ithaca: Cornell University Press, 1993); Katherine Maus, *Inwardness and Theater in the English Renaissance* (Chicago: University of Chicago Press, 1995); Jonathan Sawday, *The Body Emblazoned: Dissection and the Human Body in Renaissance Culture* (London: Routledge, 1995); David Hillman and Carla Mazzio, eds., *The Body in Parts: Fantasies of Corporeality in Early Modern Europe* (New York: Routledge, 1997); Michael Schoenfeldt, *Bodies and Selves in Early Modern England: Physiology and Inwardness in Spenser, Shakespeare, Herbert, and Milton* (Cambridge: Cambridge University Press, 1999); Valerie Traub, *The Renaissance of Lesbianism in Early Modern England* (Cambridge: Cambridge University Press, 2002); and Gail Kern Paster, *Humoring the Body: Emotions and the Shakespearean Stage* (Chicago: University of Chicago Press, 2004).

9 Gail Kern Paster, Katherine Rowe, and Mary Floyd-Wilson, eds., *Reading the Early Modern Passions: Essays in the Cultural History of Emotion* (Philadelphia: University of Pennsylvania Press, 2004).

10 Ibid., 147.

11 See Elizabeth Harvey, "Sensational Bodies, Consenting Organs: Helkiah Crooke's Incorporation of Spenser," *Spenser Studies: A Renaissance Poetry Annual* 18 (2003): 295–314.

12 Fleck's seminal work is *Genesis and Development of a Scientific Fact*, trans. Fred Bradley and Thaddeus J. Trenn (Chicago: University of Chicago Press,

1979). See also the collection of his essays and essays about his work, Robert S. Cohen and Thomas Schnelle, eds., *Cognition and Fact: Materials on Ludwik Fleck* (Dordrecht: D. Reidel Publishing Company, 1986), and especially Estephen Toulmin's essay in the volume, "Ludwik Fleck and the Historical Interpretation of Science," 267–85, to which this characterization of Fleck's thought is indebted.

13  I recognize that I am taking liberties with Fleck's terminology, which has a much more localized sense in his work than I intend here. By adapting his term, I want to point to the importance of language in gaining access to the common yet unformulated perspectives that permit writers as diverse as those I study here to engage overlapping assumptions about personhood.

14  The older argument among feminists ran roughly as follows: if femaleness is *in* the body, the norms of sex difference pervasive in our culture must really be the givens of nature rather than the fabricated impositions of a culturally constructed gender system; they are, therefore, not very susceptible to political analysis and intervention and should, therefore, be avoided. Elizabeth Wilson, Elizabeth Grosz, and others, too, reject this premise that the study of the material body cannot be enlisted in feminist projects. Wilson's most recent book, *Psychosomatic: Feminism and the Neurological Body* (Durham: Duke University Press, 2004), is a good example of this type of work. See also Elizabeth Grosz, *Volatile Bodies: Toward a Corporeal Feminism* (Bloomington: Indiana University Press, 1994).

15  Grosz, *Volatile Bodies*, ix; Wilson, *Neural Geographies: Feminism and the Microstructure of Cognition* (New York and London: Routledge, 1998), 14.

16  Wilson, *Neural Geographies*, 17.

17  Shigehisa Kuriyama, *The Expressiveness of the Body and the Divergence of Greek and Chinese Medicine* (New York: Zone Books, 1999); see chapters 3 and 4.

18  This parallel is suggested, though not pursued, by Thomas Fuchs, *The Mechanization of the Heart: Harvey and Descartes*, trans. Marjorie Grene (Rochester: University of Rochester Press, 2001), 58. In his work on animal spirits and memory, John Sutton argues even more strongly that early modern models of the self not only paralleled perceptions of the body but actually determined what was accepted biology (see *Philosophy and Memory Traces: Descartes to Connectionism* [Cambridge: Cambridge University Press, 1998]). Animal spirits faded from neurophysiological discourse, Sutton argues, less because of the accumulated effect of contradictory empirical findings than because they no longer cohered with a new self-construct that presupposed a self-conscious, responsible agent inhabiting a static body: "It came to seem that a psychophysiology which allowed cognition to rest on volatile inner fluids was incompatible with certain strong assumptions about self-agency" (220).

19  Galen, *On the Usefulness of the Parts of the Body*, trans. Margaret Tallmadge May, 2 vols. (Ithaca: Cornell University Press, 1968), 1:67 (hereafter cited as *UP*).

20  I discuss Galen's ambivalence and its implications for the Galenic notion of personhood in chapter 1.

21  For an overview of the history of
embryology, see Joseph Needham, *A
History of Embryology* (1957; repr., New
York: Arno Press, 1975). Howard Adelmann's gorgeously illustrated study
of Marcello Malpighi's life and works
has a useful overview of embryology
in the sixteenth and seventeenth centuries; see *Marcello Malpighi and the Evolution of Embryology* (Ithaca: Cornell
University Press, 1966), chapter 24. Also
see Jacques Roger, *Les sciences de la vie
dans la pensée française du XVIIIc siècle:
la génération des animaux de Descartes
à l'encyclopédie.* (Paris: Armand Collin,
1963); Elizabeth Gasking, *Investigations
into Generation, 1651–1828* (London:
Hutchinson Press, 1967); Jane Oppenheimer, *Essays in the History of Embryology and Biology* (Cambridge, Mass.: MIT
Press, 1967); and Shirley Roe, *Matter,
Life, and Generation: Eighteenth-Century
Embryology and the Haller-Wolff Debate*
(Cambridge: Cambridge University
Press, 1981).

22  Joan Cadden, *Meanings of Sex Difference*,
discusses the conflicting constructions
of medieval notions of woman (see esp.
chapter 4) and Monica Green discusses
the shift in focus in medieval gynecological medicine from woman's general
somatic constitution to her generative function; see "From 'Diseases of
Women' to 'Secrets of Women': The
Transformation of Gynecological Literature in the Later Middle Ages," *Journal of Medieval and Early Modern Studies*
30.1 (Winter, 2000): 5–39.

23  Karen Newman has demonstrated
both the pervasiveness and, ultimately,
the inadequacy of these binaries in
visual represetations of the fetus from

the seventeenth through the twenti-
eth century. For Newman, the image
of the routinely "missing" or passive
body of the reproductive woman (and
the corresponding fetal autonomy that
image assumes) not only undergirds
the emergence of the modern masculine subject, but also, and perhaps
more presssingly, sets the conceptual
limitations of the current and highly
politicized abortion debates. See *Fetal
Positions: Individualism, Science, Visuality*
(Stanford: Stanford University Press,
1996). Though Newman focuses on
visual rather than verbal constructions
of the fetus and in brief scope trav-
erses four centuries of such images,
my work, in the broad outlines of its
project—in asking after the relations
between the rhetoric of early modern
medicine and the production of a gendered and rights-bearing subject—
is indebted to Newman's important
study.

24  See, for example, Richard Jonas,
trans., *The Byrth of Mankynde, newly
translated out of Laten into Englysshe*
(London: Thomas Raynalde, 1540),
XVIIr, and Jacques Guillemeau, *Childbirth; or, the Happy Deliverie of Women*
(London: A. Hatfield, 1612), 112.

25  As Harvey says, and as I will explore
in chapter 4.

26  Clifford Geertz, "From the Native's
Point of View: On the Nature of
Anthropological Understanding,"
*Interpretive Social Science: A Reader,*
ed. R. Rabinow and W. M. Sullivan
(Berkeley: University of California
Press, 1979), 222.

27  Kuriyama, *Expressiveness of the Body*, 272.

28  Jonathan Sawday, "Self and Selfhood

in the Seventeenth Century," in Porter, *Rewriting the Self*, 30.

29  Roger Smith, "Self-Reflection and the Self," in Porter, *Rewriting the Self*, 50.

30  John Milton, *Paradise Lost* (4.486), in *John Milton: Complete Poems and Major Prose*, ed. Merritt Y. Hughes (New York: Odyssey Press, 1957).

31  The classic study of the challenge of mindful matter in the eighteenth century is John W. Yolton's *Thinking Matter: Materialism in Eighteenth-Century Britain* (Minneapolis: University of Minnesota Press, 1983).

32  G. S. Rousseau and Roy Porter, "Introduction: Toward a Natural History of Mind and Body," in *The Languages of Psyche: Mind and Body in Enlightenment Thought*, ed. G. S. Rousseau (Berkeley: University of California Press, 1990), 39.

33  Fuchs, *Mechanization of the Heart*. Fuchs demonstrates that though Harvey was profoundly indebted both to vitalism and Aristotelianism, the circulation of the blood was interpreted mechanistically in the decades following its discovery. Fuchs neatly summarizes his argument in his introduction.

34  I am thinking here of Hans Moravec, whom I discuss at greater length in chapter 1.

35  Sandra Blakeslee, "When the Brain Says, 'Don't Get Too Close,'" *New York Times* (13 July 2004), F2.

36  These questions are now routinely asked as well in the burgeoning fields of animal studies and disability studies; both struggle with the conceptual and political limitations of rights discourse. An attempt to break free from the ultimately ethical strictures of a still-entrenched humanist assumption of rights in animal studies can be found in Cary Wolfe, *Animal Rites: American Culture, the Discourse of Species, and Posthumanist Theory* (Chicago: University of Chicago Press, 2003).

37  As the next two chapters will indicate, Galenism, though ancient in origin, dominated Western medicine through the sixteenth century. I, therefore, refer to Galenism as premodern because, in its various permutations over the centuries, Galenism provided the normative framework for biomedicine up to the early modern period.

38  Rebecca Flemming argues a similar point about medicine in ancient Rome; see *Medicine and the Making of Roman Women: Gender, Nature, and Authority from Celsus to Galen* (Oxford: Oxford University Press, 2000), 1–33.

39  Bruno Latour, "Why Has Critique Run out of Steam? From Matters of Fact to Matters of Concern," *Critical Inquiry* 30 (Winter, 2004), 225–48; see esp. 231.

40  Ibid.

41  Ibid., 228.

42  Ibid., 237.

43  Ludwik Fleck, "On the Crisis of 'Reality,'" in Cohen and Schnelle, *Cognition and Fact*, 55.

44  Latour, "Why Has Critique Run out of Steam?" 246.

## *1 / On Either Side of the Early Modern: Posthuman and Premodern Bodies and Selves*

1  For a fascinating discussion of the posthuman in regenerative medicine, see Eugene Thacker, "Data Made Flesh: Biotechnology and the

Discourse of the Posthuman," *Cultural Critique* 53 (Winter, 2003): 72–97.

2 The by now classic work tracing the overlapping patterns of innovation and replication in posthumanism is N. Katherine Hayles, *How We Became Posthuman: Virtual Bodies in Cybernetics, Literature, and Informatics* (Chicago: University of Chicago Press, 1999). See also the collection of essays included in *Cultural Critique* 53 (Winter, 2003).

3 Patricia Smith Churchland, *Brain-Wise: Studies in Neurophilosohpy* (Cambridge, Mass.: MIT Press, 2002), 25.

4 Moravec is the founder of the robotics institute at Carnegie Mellon University. He first proposed the possible downloading of consciousness into silicon in *Mind Children: The Future of Robot and Human Intelligence* (Cambridge, Mass.: Harvard University Press, 1988), and he has developed the argument concerning the theoretical reach of robotic intelligence in his more recent book, *Robot: Mere Machine to Transcendent Mind* (New York: Oxford University Press, 1999).

5 Hayles, *How We Became Posthuman*, 5.

6 Rodney Brooks, *Flesh and Machines: How Robots Will Change Us* (New York: Pantheon Books, 2002), 22. For an assessment of Brooks's work in the evolution of AI and robotic intelligence, see John Johnston, "A Future for Autonomous Agents: Machinic *Merkwelten* and Artificial Evolution," *Configurations* 10.3 (2002): 473–517.

7 Brooks, *Flesh and Machines*, 38.

8 Ibid., 46.

9 One such mobile robot that Brooks describes is Shakey, built at Stanford in the late 1960s and early 1970s.

Shakey, which was "about the size of a small adult," was able to move through several rooms and push particular colored blocks from one room to another as it followed commands slowly calculated by its physically separate mainframe computer. The mainframe computer, Brooks explains, "did the thinking and sent commands back to its physical avatar, the shell of a robot, in the physical world" (ibid., 22).

10 Ibid., 94

11 See Donna J. Haraway, *Simians, Cyborgs, and Women: The Reinvention of Nature* (New York: Routledge, 1991); Francisco J. Varela, Evan Thompson, and Eleanor Rosch, *The Embodied Mind: Cognitive Science and Human Experience* (Cambridge, Mass.: MIT Press, 1991); and Grosz, *Volatile Bodies*.

12 See A. R. Damasio, *The Feeling of What Happens: Body and Emotion in the Making of Consciousness* (New York: Harcourt Brace, 1999), 14, for a list of some of the technologies that make it possible to observe real-time correlation between mental and neural events.

13 These traditionally philosophical questions are addressed by, among others, Patricia Churchland, *Neurophilosophy: Towards a Unified Understanding of the Mind-Brain* (Cambridge, Mass.: MIT Press, 1986); Gerald Edelman, *Bright Air, Brilliant Fire: On the Matter of Mind* (New York: Basic Books, 1992); V. S. Ramachandran and Sandra Blakesless, *Phantoms in the Brain: Probing the Mysteries of the Human Mind* (New York: William Morrow, 1998); Damasio, *The Feeling of What Happens*; Churchland, *Brain-Wise*; and Owen Flanagan, *The*

*Problem of the Soul: Two Visions of Mind and How to Reconcile Them* (New York: Basic Books, 2002). Damasio himself remarks how questionable it was considered until recently to attempt a neurological analysis of consciousness: "Studying consciousness was simply not the thing to do before you made tenure, and even after you did it was looked upon with suspicion. Only in recent years has consciousness become a somewhat safer topic of scientific inquiry" (*The Feeling of What Happens,* 7). In outlining some of the ways in which questions of selfhood are now pursued empirically, I do not mean to suggest that brain science provides a value-neutral ground on which to build answers to these questions, though some brain researchers themselves may think that. My purpose here is not to evaluate the social construction of modern brain research; rather, it is to survey its suggestions about the construction and nature of consciousness and the self.

14  Churchland, *Brain-Wise*, 270.

15  For various voices skeptical of the usefulness of neurological research to questions of mind, see Paul Churchland, *Matter and Consciousness,* rev. ed. (Cambridge, Mass.: MIT Press, 1988), 144; Owen Flanagan, *The Science of the Mind*, 2nd ed. (Cambridge, Mass.: MIT Press, 1991), 307ff.; Churchland, *Brain-Wise*, 154; and see Thomas Nagel, "What Is it Like to Be a Bat?," *Mortal Questions* (Cambridge: Cambridge University Press, 1979) for one of the now classic arguments against the ability of empirical science to capture the subjective phenomenon of consciousness.

16  Churchland, *Brain-Wise*, 20–29.

17  Quoted in Flanagan, *The Problem of the Soul*, 176.

18  Ibid., 177.

19  The example is Churchland's. See Churchland, *Brain-Wise*, 59–63.

20  See Damasio, *The Feeling of What Happens*, 134, and Churchland, *Brain-Wise*, 59ff.

21  Damasio defines the proto-self as follows: "The proto-self is a coherent collection of neural patterns which map, moment by moment, the state of the physical structure of the organism in its many dimensions" (*The Feeling of What Happens*, 155). See also Churchland, *Brain-Wise*, 71ff.

22  The fundamental distinction Damasio draws between core and autobiographical selves is a temporal one: the self that emerges from what Damasio calls "core consciousness" is transient, recreated on a moment-by-moment basis as the brain interacts with an object; the autobiographical self, which emerges from what Damasio calls "extended consciousness," provides the sense of self that is consistent over time, that is aware of both past and future. Damasio employs these concepts in all his books, but he discusses them at greatest length in *The Feeling of What Happens*. See especially chapters 3, 6, and 7.

23  Damasio, *The Feeling of What Happens*, 116.

24  Churchland, *Brain-Wise*, 71.

25  Flanagan, *The Science of the Mind*, 207.

26  Churchland, *Brain-Wise*, 44.

27  Ibid., 46.

28  On the correspondences between neurological damage and neuropsycho-

logical deficits see Paul Churchland, *Matter and Consciousness*, 143; Gerald Edelman, and Giulio Tononi, *A Universe of Consciousness: How Matter Becomes Imagination* (New York: Basic Books, 2000), 28; and Patricia Churchland, *Brain-Wise*, 64. In the tradition of Oliver Sacks, Ramachandran, *Phantoms in the Brain*, and Damasio, *The Feeling of What happens*, also offer philosophically inflected case histories of individuals with such conditions.

29 Edelman sets out his theory both in *Bright Air, Brilliant Fire* and, with Giulio Tononi, in *A Universe of Consciousness*.

30 Andy Clark, *Natural-Born Cyborgs: Minds, Technologies, and the Future of Human Intelligence* (New York: Oxford University Press, 2003), 10.

31 Ibid., 42.

32 Ibid., 138–39.

33 Flanagan, *The Problem of the Soul*, xii.

34 The standard version of the history of Galenism in the West is Oswei Temkin, *Galenism: Rise and Decline of a Medical Philosophy* (Ithaca: Cornell University Press, 1973). See also Luis García-Ballester, *Galen and Galenism: Theory and Medical Practice from Antiquity to the European Renaissance*, Jon Arrizabalaga, Montserrat Cabré, Lluís Cifuentes, Fernando Salmón, eds. (Burlington, VT: Ashgate, 2002), a collection of essays (in English, Spanish, and German) devoted both to Galen's life and times and to the legacy of Galenism, especially in the Latin West. For discussions of some of Galen's treatises not included in Karl Gottlob Kühn and F. W. Assmann's nineteenth-century edition *Opera Omnia*, 22 vols. (Leipzig: C. Cnobloch, 1821–1833) see Vivian Nut-

ton, ed., *The Unknown Galen* (London: University of London, 2002). For an excellent and focused discussion of women in Galen's works, see Flemming, *Medicine and the Making of Roman Women*.

35 Because my purpose here is schematic, and because I am working from modern English translations of Galen's texts, I do not generally rely on the same kind of rhetorical close reading in my analysis here as I do in other chapters. I mean to sketch a model detailed enough to highlight broad overlaps between Galen's understanding of the self and posthumanism, which can serve in subsequent chapters as norms against which I will read the rhetorical formulations of early modern writers.

36 In proposing these areas of overlap between Galen and the posthuman, I am of course eliding numerous variations in western understandings of self and body that emerge over the centuries up to the early modern period. To mention just a few examples: Cicero (106–43 BCE) understood the injunction "know thyself" as a call to know one's soul, separate and distinct from the body; for Augustine (CE 354–430), the call to know one's self meant recognizing the individual soul's essential connection to the divine. Arguably, for these writers, as surely for others, the self *was* in some sense disembodied. But it was not disembodied *in the same way* as it came to be in the early modern and modern periods; it was not an autonomous essence and it was not separable, conceptually or ontologically, from the sociopolitical or

divinely endowed contexts in which it existed. Augustine may have written of something we might think of as interiority, but it was a specifically Christian interiority, one that found its essence in its bond with God, not in the particularities and vagaries of an isolated and individual mind. Even Petrarch, so often heralded as the harbinger of modern individualism, does not fit the modern mold. As Timothy Reiss puts it: "Not for him the belief in a Dignity of Man pitted alone against Nature and Fortune, responsible for his own Fate, ennobled by Promethean individualism. Not for him even modest belief in humans as essentially characterized by 'interiority.'" That these are variations on rather than clear breaks from ancient assumptions is the central premise of Timothy J. Reiss's book, *Mirages of the Selfe: Patterns of Personhood in Ancient and Early Modern Europe.* (Stanford: Stanford University Press, 2003), 303; also see chapters 4 and 9.

37  Galen, *On the Natural Faculties*, trans. and ed., Arthur John Brock (London: Hienemann, 1916), 9 (hereafter cited in text at *NF*).

38  Reiss, *Mirages of the Selfe*, 220.

39  Ibid., 2.

40  Ibid., emphasis mine.

41  Though translated as "soul," the term *psyche*, for reasons that should become clear, does not convey in Greek medicine the sense of opposition to the body that it generally does in Christian culture. Several essays treating psyche and soma in the ancient world, along with excellent bibliographies on the topic, may be found in John P. Wright and Paul Potter, eds., *Psyche and Soma: Physicians and Metaphysicians on the Mind-Body Problem from Antiquity to Enlightenment* (Oxford: Clarendon Press, 2000).

42  It hardly needs saying that, nearly 2,000 years later, this question of correlation remains unresolved.

43  Galen, *Opera Omnia*, ed. Karl Gottlob Kühn, 22 vols. (Leipzig: Carolus Cnoblochius, 1821–1833), IV.700–2; quoted on page 202 in R. James Hankinson, "Galen's Anatomy of the Soul," *Phronesis* 36.2 (1991): 197–233.

44  Luis García-Ballester, "Soul and Body: Disease of the Soul and Disease of the Body in Galen's Medical Thought," in P. Manuli and M. Vegetti, eds., *Le opere psicologiche de Galeno* (Naples: Bibliopolis, 1988), 136.

45  Galen, *Opera Omnia*, IV.577; quoted in Hankinson, "Galen's Anatomy of the Soul," 229.

46  Galen, "The Soul's Dependence on the Body" in *Galen: Selected Works*, trans. and ed. P. N. Singer (Oxford: Oxford University Press), 159–60.

47  Ibid., 167–68.

48  Galen, *On the Doctrines of Hippocrates and Plato*, (trans. and ed. Phillip De Lacy), 3 vols. (Berlin: Akademie-Verlag, 1978–1984), 2.445.

49  Quoted in García-Ballester, "Soul and Body," 150.

50  On Galen's theories of brain function and his numerous experiments to demonstrate that the brain was the seat of the rational soul, see Julius Rocca, *Galen on the Brain: Anatomical Knowledge and Physiological Speculation in the Second Century* (Leiden, Boston: Brill, 2003).

51 Elizabeth Wilson attests to this same discomfort, really, this inability to conceptualize a thoroughgoing psychosomatology, in her work on current research in and evaluations of the enteric nervous system. Wilson shows how, despite evidence suggesting, literally, a "psychology of the gut," and despite an awareness that the psyche is frequently a factor in disturbances of the gut, current bio-medical literature cannot conceptualize adequately how the psyche and the gut relate: "One way or another, most . . . commentators try to keep psychology at a distance from the gut" (*Psychosomatics*, 39).

52 Hankinson, "Galen's Anatomy of the Soul," 229–30.

53 R. J. Hankinson, "Actions and Passions: Affection, Emotion, and Moral Self-Management in Galen's Philosophical Psychology," in Jacques Brunschwig and Martha C. Nussbaum, ed., *Passions and Perceptions: Studies in Hellenistic Philosophy of Mind* (Cambridge: Cambridge University Press, 1993), 192–93.

54 Hayles, *How We Became Posthuman*, 3.

55 Ibid., 6.

56 Hillman and Mazzio, eds. *The Body in Parts*.

57 Wallace I. Matson, "Why Isn't the Mind-Body Problem Ancient?" in Paul Feyerabend and Grover Maxwell, eds., *Mind, Matter, and Method: Essays in Philosophy and Science in Honor of Herbert Feigl* (Minneapolis: University of Minnesota Press, 1966), 97. In brief scope, Matson explicates the assumption of mind-body identity in Greek thought, particularly in contrast to more current concerns about the mind-body relation as a problem.

## 2 / Subjectified Parts and Supervnient Selves: Rewriting Galenism in Crooke's Microcosmographia

1 On Renaissance editions of Galen, see R. J. Durling, "A Chronological Census of Renaissance Editions and Translations of Galen," *Journal of the Warburg and Cortauld Institute* 24 (1961): 230–305.

2 This is not to suggest that Galen did not exist in the Latin West in the earlier Middle Ages; some Galenic material was preserved in Latin compilations and through post-Galenic writers like Nemesius and Oribasius. See Temkin's survey of the rise and fall of Galenism in the West in *Galenism: Rise and Decline*.

3 For an overview of medieval medical education and the role of Galenism in its structure and content, see Nancy G. Siraisi, *Medieval and Early Renaissance Medicine: An Introduction to Knowledge and Practice* (Chicago: University of Chicago Press, 1990), esp. chapter 3.

4 Jo. Manardus, *Epistolarum Medicinalium*, 1535, 13, quoted in Andrew Wear, "Galen in the Renaissance," in *Galen: Problems and Prospects*, ed. Vivian Nutton, (London: The Wellcome Institute for the History of Medicine, 1981), 230.

5 On English medical humanists, see Vivian Nutton, *John Caius and the Manuscripts of Galen* (Cambridge: Cambridge Philological Society, 1987); Charles David O'Malley, *English Medical Humanists: Thomas Linacre and John Caius* (Lawrence: University of Kansas Press,

1965); and Francis Maddison, Margaret Pelling, and Charles Webster, eds., *Essays on the Life and Work of Thomas Linacre, c. 1460–1524* (Oxford: The Clarendon Press, 1977).

6 K. F. Russell determined that by 1600, 150 medical books written in English appeared in close to 400 editions; see "A Checklist of Medical Books Published in English before 1600," *Bulletin of the History of Medicine* 21 (1947): 922–58. Charles Webster determined that of the 238 medical books published in England between 1640 and 1660, only thirty-one appeared in Latin; see *The Great Instauration: Science, Medicine, and Reform, 1626–1660* (London: Duckworth, 1975), 259. These data, compiled decades ago, underestimate the number of medical books published in English. The online English Short Title Catalogue, because it consistently adds previously unrecorded books to its list, provides the most up-to-date information. On medical book publishing in early modern England generally, see Elizabeth Furdell, *Publishing and Medicine in Early Modern England* (Rochester: University of Rochester Press, 2002). On the vernacularization of medical learning in England, see Paul Slack, "Mirrors of Health and Treasures of Poor Men: The Uses of the Vernacular Medical Litearture of Tudor England," in *Health, Medicine and Mortality in the Sixteenth Century*, ed., Charles Webster (Cambridge: Cambridge University Press, 1979), 237–73, and the essays collected in Roy Porter, ed., *The Popularization of Medicine, 1650–1750* (London: Routledge, 1992).

7 Crooke writes within a predominantly Galenic paradigm even about issues relating to the female reproductive body. The Latin and Greek editions of the Hippocratic corpus were published in 1525 and 1526, respectively, and they included the three Hippocratic works specifically devoted to what we would call gynecology, namely, *Diseases of Women, On Sterile Women*, and *Nature of Woman*. But Galen had always presented himself as following in the tradition established by Hippocrates, and, as both Helen King and Vivian Nutton have shown, Hippocrates's works tended to be read in Galenic terms through the sixteenth century. My interest here (and in the rest of the book) is therefore on variations of the Galenic, as opposed to the strictly Hippocratic, models of the body. For an excellent collection of essays on the uses and re-imaginings of Hippocrates following the publication of the Hippocratic corpus in the sixteenth century, see David Cantor, ed., *Reinventing Hippocrates* (Aldershot: Ashgate, 2002), especially Helen King, "The Power of Paternity: The Father of Medicine Meets the Prince of Physicians." See also Vivian Nutton, "Hippocrates in the Renaissance," in *Die Hippokratischen Epidemien: Theorie—Praxis—Tradition: Verhandlungen des Ve Colloque International Hippocratique, Sudhoffs Archiv Beiheft* 27 (1989): 420–39.

8 Helkiah Crooke, *Microcosmographia: A Description of the Body of Man* (London: William Jaggard, 1615), 2 (hereafter cited as *M*).

9   Addressing the barber-surgeons as he calls them, and clearly thinking of an audience both interested in and able to afford so weighty a text, Crooke was surely not writing in order to attract patients to his practice as an unlicensed "irregular" might. But the relative authority of surgeons versus physicians was at issue for him, as I hope to show, and, in that sense, he was engaged in the competitive market of early modern medicine. On the competition between physicians and surgeons, see Cook, *Decline of the Old Medical Regime*, and Wear, *Knowledge and Practice*, chapter 5.

10  On sixteenth- and seventeenth-century efforts to distinguish surgeons from empirics, see Wear, *Knowledge and Practice*, chapter 5.

11  I will explore the role that this distinction between manual and rational labor would come to play in the establishment of male midwifery and obstetrics in chapter 6.

12  John Banister, *The Historie of Man* (London: John Daye, 1578), B1 r (hereafter cited as *HM*).

13  John Securis, *A Detection and Querimonie of the Daily Enormities and Abuses Comitted in Physick* (London: T. Marsh, 1566), B1r-v. For more on Securis, a Salisbury physician, see Wear, *Knowledge and Practice*, 218–20.

14  Wear, *Knowledge and Practice*, chapter 10.

15  On the Royal College of Physicians, see George N. Clark, *A History of the Royal College of Physicians*, 2 vols. (Oxford: Clarendon Press, 1964–1966). More recently, and particularly on the College's dealings with irregu-

lar practitioners, see Pelling, *Medical Conflicts in Early Modern London*.

16  In chapter 3, I discuss the particular problem of translating women's medical material into the vernacular.

17  Thomas Elyot, *The Castel of Health*, 1541, facsimile edition (New York: Scholar's Facsimilies, 1936), A2r, and A4r–v.

18  Nicholas Culpeper, *Culpeper's School of Physic* (London: N. Brook, 1659), 401. I will discuss Culpeper at greater length in chapter 3.

19  Charles David O'Malley, "Helkiah Crooke, M.D., P.R.C.P, 1576–1648," *Bulletin of the History of Medicine* 42.1 (1968), 7–8.

20  Furdell, *Publishing and Medicine in Early Modern England*, argues that the incentive to publish medical books in the vernacular was almost entirely financial rather than political, and that the correlation between radical political affiliations of booksellers and the kinds of books they published was incidental. See esp. chapter 1.

21  *Microcosmographia* is heavily indebted to these two authors who were prominent continental anatomists of the time, and in many places Crooke's text is simply a translation of their works. Crooke is altogether up front about his indebtedness, even indicating on the title pages that his material is "collected and translated out of all the best Authors of Anatomy, especially out of Casper Bauhin and Andreas Laurentius." Crooke adds in the preface that he changed the wording where he thought necessary and added the summaries at the beginning of each of the books.

22  See Sawday, both *Body Emblazoned*,

chapter 1, and "Self and Selfhood in the Seventeenth Century," in Porter, *Rewriting the Self*, 29–49, for the conceptual connections between anatomy and autopsy, or self-seeing.

23 On early Christian discomfort with Galen's materialism, see Reiss, *Mirages of the Selfe*, 224f., and Temkin, *Galenism: Rise and Decline*, 84f.

24 Temkin, *Galenism: Rise and Decline*, 78.

25 Andreas Vesalius, *De humani corporis fabrica libri septem* (Basileoe: ex officina Ioannis Oporini, 1543). On the history of the *rete mirabile* and current speculation about its function in animals that do possess it, see John Forrester, "The Marvellous Network and the History of Enquiry into its Function," *Journal of the History of Medicine and Allied Sciences* 57.2 (2002): 198–217.

26 Hillman and Mazzio, *The Body in Parts*, xiv.

27 Thomas Laqueur first popularized both the concept and the phrase, "one-sex model," though he has been taken to task for exaggerating its ubiquity both in the ancient world and in the Renaissance. For critiques of Laqueur's work, see note 7 to the introduction here.

28 On ancient debates about the status of the womb as a living thing or a wild animal, see Helen King, "Once upon a Text: The Hippocratic Origins of Hysteria," in *Hysteria Beyond Freud*, eds., Sander Gilman, Helen King, Roy Porter, G.S. Rousseau, and Elaine Showalter (Berkeley: University of California Press, 1993).

29 William Whately, *A Bride-Bush, or A Vvedding Sermon* (London: William Iaggard, 1617), 214.

30 In seventeenth-century literature, Milton's *Paradise Lost* perhaps best exemplifies the tension between a woman's self-directedness and the need for that self to be directed to the patriarchal order. Mary Nyquist offers a good analysis of this tension in "The Genesis of Gendered Subjectivity in the Divorce Tracts and in *Paradise Lost*," in *Re-Membering Milton: Essays on the Texts and Traditions*, eds., Mary Nyquist and Margaret Furgeson (New York: Metheun, 1987), 99–127.

31 See Mary Fissell, "Gender and Generation: Representing Reproduction in Early Modern England," *Gender and History* 7.3 (1995): 433–56 for a discussion of contemporary connotations of the names given to female reproductive anatomy in vernacular biomedical texts.

## 3 / Fixing the Female: Books of Practical Physic for Women

1 John Sadler, *The Sicke Womans Private Looking-Glasse* (London: Anne Griffin), 1636.

2 Nicholas Sudell, *Mulierum amicus: Or, the Womans Friend* (London: J. Hancock, 1666), A2r (hereafter cited as *MA*).

3 On early modern English medical literature for women, see Audrey Eccles, *Obstetrics and Gynecology in Tudor and Stuart England* (Kent, Ohio: Kent State University Press, 1982); Robert Erickson, "The Books of Generation: Some Observations on the Style of the English Midwife Books, 1671–1764," in *Sexuality in Eighteenth-Century Britain*, ed. Paul-Gabriel Boucé (Manchester: Manchester University Press, 1982),

79–94; and several works by Mary Fissell, including "Readers, Texts, and Contexts: Vernacular Medical Works in Early Modern England," in *Popularization of Medicine*, ed. Roy Porter; "Gender and Generation"; "Making a Masterpiece: The *Aristotle* Texts in Medical Culture," in *Right Living: An Anglo-American Tradition of Self-Help Medicine and Hygiene*, ed. Charles E. Rosenberg (Baltimore: Johns Hopkins University Press, 2003). See also Elaine Hobby's introduction to her edition of Jane Sharp's *The Midwives Book, or the Whole Art of Midwifry Discovered* (New York: Oxford University Press, 1999 [1671]).

4 On the common areas of interest that began to emerge in late-medieval studies of generation and sex difference, see Cadden, *Meanings of Sex Difference*, chapters 2 and 3.

5 Ibid., 170f.

6 For medieval assessments of the menses, see Cadden, *Meanings of Sex Difference*, 170ff., and Carole Rawcliffe, *Medicine and Society in Later Medieval England* (Phoenix Mill: Sutton Publishing, 1997), 175. . On opinions about menstruation in the Renaissance, see Patricia Crawford, "Attitudes to Menstruation in Seventeenth-Century England," *Past and Present* 91 (1981): 47–73.

7 Cadden, *Meanings of Sex Difference*, 178; Newman, *Fetal Positions*, 33.

8 Thomas Raynalde, trans., *The Byrth of Mankynde*, by Eucharius Rösslin (London, 1545), 45r and 44r (hereafter cited as *R.BM*). (Throughout, I have preserved original spellings but have silently expanded abbreviated words.)

9 Webster, *Great Instauration*, 267; Furdell, *Publishing and Medicine in Early Modern England*, 35. See also the sources listed in chapter 2, note 6 here.

10 On the popularization of medical literature in the early modern period, see Andrew Wear, "Popularization of Medicine in Early Modern England," as well as the other articles in Porter, *Popularization of Medicine*. Chapter 4 of Wear's *Knowledge and Practice* also discusses the widespread dissemination of vernacular health advice books in early modern culture.

11 For an analysis of Wolveridge's manual, particularly in contrast to the first midwifery guide written in English by a woman, Jane Sharp's *The Midwives Book*, see Eve Keller, "Mrs. Jane Sharp: Midwifery and the Critique of Medical Knowledge in Seventeenth-Century England," *Women's Writing* 2.2 (1995):101–111.

12 Sadler, *The Sicke Womans Private Looking-Glasse*, 55–56.

13 Nicholas Culpeper, *A Directory for Midwives, or A Guide for Women*, 2nd ed. (London: Peter Cole, 1656), 76 (hereafter cited as *DM*).

14 Richard Jonas, *The Byrth of Mankynde, newly translated out of Laten into Englyshe* (London: Thomas Raynalde, 1540) (hereafter cited as *J.BM*). For a reading of the first two editions of *Byrth* in the context of the contested religious connotations of conception, pregnancy, and birth, see Fissell, *Vernacular Bodies*, 29–35.

15 On the printing history of *The Byrth of Mankynde* along with a comparative analysis of its contents among its many editions, see J. W. Ballantyne,

*"The Byrth of Mankynde*: Its Author and Editions," *The Journal of Obstetrics and Gynaecology of the British Empire* 10.4 (1906): 297–326 and *"The Byrth of Mankynde*: Its Contents," *The Journal of Obstetrics and Gynaecology of the British Empire* 12.3 (1907): 175–94 and 12.4 (1907): 255–74.

16  Monica Green, "Obstetrical and Gynaecological Texts in Middle English," *Studies in the Age of Chaucer* 14 (1992), 58. Compare, too, the English translator of Jacques Guillemeau's French text on midwifery, who hopes that he has not "been offensive to Women, in prostituting and divulging that, which they would not have come to open light, and which beside cannot be exprest in such proper terms, as are fit for the virginitie of pen and paper, and the white sheetes of the Child-bed" (Guillemeau, *Child-birth or, The Happy Deliuerie of Vvomen* [London: A. Hatfield, 1612], jj2 v). The translator worries typically about divulging women's secrets and thereby defiling the purity of what is best kept hidden, but he does not worry about the act of reading, about the open-endedness of interpretation, as Raynalde does here.

17  Though the two-seed model of conception was a commonplace in Galenic medicine, the so-called one-sex model on which it was based was not universally accepted. See Winfried Schleiner, "Early Modern Controversies about the One-Sex Model," *Renaissance Quarterly* 53.1 (2000): 180–91 for an overview of the debates.

18  For a detailed analysis of the conceptualization of woman in Galen and in Roman medicine generally, see Flem-

ming, *Medicine and the Making of Roman Women.*

19  After the mid-seventeenth century, midwifery manuals started to appear in great numbers; by the end of the century, the most common were the *Aristotle's Masterpiece* books, which were, really, more popular guides to sex, pregnancy, and childbirth than midwifery manuals per se. See especially Mary Fissell, "Hairy Women and Naked Truths: Gender and the Politics of Knowledge in *Aristotle's Masterpiece,*" *William and Mary Quarterly* 60.1 (January, 2003): 43–74 and "Making a Masterpiece"; see also Roy Porter and Lesley Hall, *The Facts of Life: The Creation of Sexual Knowledge in Britain, 1650–1950* (New Haven: Yale University Press, 1995).

20  On Culpeper generally, see F. N. L. Poynter, "Nicholas Culpeper and his Books," *Journal of the History of Medicine* 17 (1962): 152–67 and "Nicholas Culpeper and the Paracelsians," in *Science, Medicine, and Society in the Renaissance: Essays to Honor Walter Pagel*, 2 vols., ed. Allen G. Debus (New York: American Elsevier Press, 1972): 1.201–220, from which the biographical information included here is drawn. There is also a biographical sketch, presumably written by Culpeper's amanuensis, in *Culpeper's School of Physic* (London: N. Brook, 1659). Olav Thulesius's biography, *Nicholas Culpeper: English Physician and Astrologer* (New York: St. Martin's Press, 1992), is more impressionistic than scholarly but gives a lively sense of Culpeper's work as herbalist and astrologer. Fissell, *Vernacular Bodies*, chapter 5, offers an inci-

sive treatment of Culpeper's works in the context of the polarized politics of Civil War London and of the particular upheavals in gender hierarchy that the period produced.

21  He also apparently left his wife scores of unpublished manuscripts, which she sold after his death to support herself.

22  Nicholas Culpeper, *A Physicall Directory, or, A Translation of the London Dispensatory* (London: Peter Cole, 1649), A1r.

23  I question the sincerity of the invitation to correction because it seems more a rhetorical strategy to win a woman reader's confidence than a genuine openness to improvement. After all, he writes to instruct women in what they already practice, a practice in which he has no experience, and he routinely grounds his claim to superior knowledge on having seen dissections which, presumably, most midwives would not have had access to.

24  By the mid-seventeenth century, when most of these books were published, Galenic medicine was increasingly challenged by the growing popularity of chemical medicine. But my focus here remains on more or less traditional Galenic medicine, both because that remained the most prevalent form of professional medicine through the end of the century and because most of the texts on women's healthcare continued to promote it. For changes and continuities in medical practice in the later part of the seventeenth century, see Wear, *Knowledge and Practice*, chapter 10.

25  Lazarus Riverius, *The Practice of Physicke*, "by" Nicholas Culpeper, Abdiah Cole, William Rowland (London: George Sawbridge,1678), 417 (hereafter cited as *PP*).

26  On seventeenth-century reevaluations of the etiology of hysteria, especially Syndenham's delocalizing of the condition from the womb and Willis's shifting it to a dysfunction of the nerves, see Jeffrey Boss, "The Seventeenth-Century Transformation of the Hysteric Affection, and Sydenham's Baconian Medicine," *Psychological Medicine* 9 (1979): 221–34; and Robert Martenson, "'The Transformation of Eve': Women's Bodies, Medicine, and Culture in Early Modern England," in *Sexual Knowledge, Sexual Science: The History of Attitudes to Sexuality*, ed. Roy Porter and Mikulás Teich (Cambridge: Cambridge University Press, 1997), 107–34; on hysteria more generally in early modern Europe, see G. S. Rousseau, "'A Strange Pathology': Hysteria in the Early Modern World, 1500–1800," in *Hysteria Beyond Freud*, ed. Sander Gilman, Helen King, Roy Porter, G. S. Rousseau, and Elaine Showalter (Berkeley: University of California Press, 1993), 91–225; on hysteria in the ancient world, see King, "Once upon a Text."

27  Edward Jorden, *A Briefe Discourse of a Disease Called the Suffocation of the Mother* (London: John Windet, 1603), 2r (hereafter cited as *BD*). Jorden wrote his book following his involvement in the celebrated trial of an accused witch. In 1602, Mary Glover, suddenly blind, inarticulate, and suffering from some kind of fits, was thought by

some to be suffering from "suffocation of the mother"; others thought she was possessed by demons. An older acquaintance with whom Glover had had some unpleasant dealings was put on trial for witchcraft and Jorden was one of two doctors who testified at the trial that the cause of Glover's ailment was natural rather than supernatural. His twenty-seven-page pamphlet came out one year later. For details of the case, editions of the central pamphlets published in connection with it, and an analysis of the religious and political issues it involved, see Michael MacDonald, *Witchcraft and Hysteria in Elizabethan London: Edward Jorden and the Mary Glover Case* (London: Tavistock/Routledge, 1991).

28 Sadler voices the same belief, ultimately Hippocratic in origin, that the womb is the central cause of disease in women. As he says in his introduction, "When I had spent some meditations, and consulted with Galen and Hippocrates for my proceeding; amongst all diseases incident to the body, I found none more frequent, none more perilous then those which arise from the ill affected wombe: for through the evil quality thereof, the heart, the liver, and the braine are affected" (Sadler, *Sicke Womans,* A4v).

## 4 / Making Up for Losses: The Workings of Gender in Harvey's De generatione animalium

1 William Harvey, *Anatomical Exercitations, Concerning the Generation of Living Creatures* (London: James Young, 1653) a5r (hereafter cited as *DG*, abbreviated

from its Latin title, *De generatione animalium,* since the treatise is generally referred to by that name). It is not known who made the translation, though it is often thought to be by Dr. Ent, who initially urged Harvey to publish the treatise. See Geoffrey Keynes, *The Life of William Harvey* (Oxford: Clarendon Press, 1966), 336–37. The 1653 edition, though less mellifluous than the 1847 translation by Robert Willis, is much more faithful to the original text.

2 For discussions of Harvey's embryology, see A. W. Meyer, *An Analysis of the "De generatione" of William Harvey* (Stanford: Stanford University Press, 1936), which is devoted exclusively to Harvey's text and quotes extensively from nineteenth- and twentieth-century scholars. See also Walter Pagel's two still standard works, *William Harvey's Biological Ideas: Selected Aspects and Historical Background* (New York: Hafner, 1967) and *New Light on William Harvey* (Basel: Karger, 1978), which treat Harvey's vitalism and his ongoing indebtedness to Aristotle. See also Elizabeth Gasking, *Investigations into Generation, 1651–1828* (London: Hutchinson, 1967), 16–37.

3 For a discussion of the history of the analogy between body and state, see Leonard Barkan, *Nature's Work of Art: The Human Body as Image of the World* (New Haven: Yale University Press, 1975).

4 Walter Charleton, *Natural History of Nutrition, Life, and Voluntary Motion* (London: Henry Herringman, 1659), A3v; quoted in John Rogers, *The Matter of Revolution: Science, Poetry, and Poli-*

*tics in the Age of Milton* (Ithaca: Cornell University Press, 1996), 19. On Harrington, see Bernard I. Cohen, "Harrington and Harvey: A Theory of the State Based on the New Physiology," *Journal of the History of Ideas* 55 (1994): 187–210. These examples of the overlap between the body and the body politic are drawn from Rogers, *Matter of Revolution*, 23–27.

5  See Rogers, *Matter of Revolution*, chapter 1.

6  William Harvey, *The Anatomical Exercises of Dr. William Harvey, De Motu Cordis: De Circulatione Sanguinis* 1649: *The First English Text of* 1653, ed. Geoffrey Keynes (London: Nonesuch, 1928), viii.

7  ibid., vii.

8  Ibid., 115. For a debate about the importance of the resonance between Harvey's physiological proposals and the reigning political philosophies of the mid-seventeenth century, see Christopher Hill, "William Harvey and the Idea of Monarchy," and Gweneth Whitteridge, "William Harvey: A Royalist and No Parliamentarian," both in *The Intellectual Revolution of the Seventeenth Century*, ed. Charles Webster (London: Routledge, 1974), 160–81 and 182–88. See also Rogers, *Matter of Revolution*, 16–38.

9  See the sources cited in the previous note.

10  Quoted in Rogers, *Matter of Revolution*, 20.

11  Thomas Fuchs, *Mechanization*, also discusses the vitalist underpinnings even of Harvey's most "mechanical" formulations.

12  Harvey took advantage of the King's passion for hunting; his stock of animals provided Harvey with material for dissection. As Harvey explained, the King's hunt was "especially the Buck and Doe; no Prince in Europe having greater store either wandring at liberty in the Woods, or Forrests, or inclosed and kept up in Parks and Chaces. In the three summer months, the Buck and Stagge were his game, and the Doe and Hind in the Autumne, and Winter, so long as the three seasonable moneths continued. Here upon (for the Rutting time, when the Females are lusty, and admit the Males, whereby they conceive and bear their young) I had a daily opportunity of dissecting them, and of making inspection and observation of all their parts; which liberty I chiefly made use of in order to the Genital parts" (*DG*, 396–97).

13  On the theory of patriarchalism, see Gordon Schochet, *Patriarchalism in Political Thought: The Authoritarian Family and Political Speculation and Attitudes, Especially in Seventeenth-Century England* (New York: Basic Books, 1975). Schochet was among the first to study at length the relations between familial and political power in seventeenth-century England, what he calls "the theory of the familial basis of politics" (5). For Schochet, patriarchalism is both a network of ideas about the divinely ordained and analogous status of a father's and a king's rule and an articulation of what existed in practice in the Stuart family, that "householders ruled their dependents with absolute authority" (57). Not all scholars have endorsed Schochet's sense of the unmitigated authority of

the patriarch; see, for example, Margaret Ezell (*The Patriarch's Wife: Literary Evidence and the History of the Family* [Chapel Hill: University of North Carolina Press, 1987]), who finds a place for female empowerment even within early modern patriarchy. See also Carole Pateman, *The Sexual Contract* (Stanford: Stanford University Press, 1988) and Rachel Weil, *Political Passions: Gender, the Family, and Political Argument in England, 1680–1714* (Manchester: Manchester University Press, 1999), discussed also in note 21, below.

14   Quoted in Schochet, *Partriarchalism*, 87.

15   Richard Field, *Of the Church,* quoted in Schochet, *Partriarchalism*, 95.

16   In his defense of the divine right of kings, Royalist John Maxwell similarly demonstrated the origin of sovereignty in Adam's rule over Eve by recalling her origin in him. "Is it not considerable that God did not make Evah out of the earth, as he did Adam, but made her *of the man*; and declareth too, made her *for him*? It is far more probably then, [that] God in his wisedome did not thinke fit . . . to make *two independents*, and liked best of all governments of mankind, *The Soveraignty of one*, and that with that extent, that both wife and posterity should submit and subject themselves to him." John Maxwell, *Sacra-Santa Regnum Majestas; or, The Sacred and Royall Prerogative of Christian Kings* (Oxford: Henry Hall, 1644), 16.

17   Sir Robert Filmer, "Observations Concerning the Original of Government," in *Sir Robert Filmer: Patriarcha and Other Writings*, ed. Johann P. Sommerville (Cambridge: Cambridge University Press, 1991), 187–88. On Filmer's use of Adamic paternity to ground his argument for absolute monarchy in another of his works, *The Anarchy of a Limited or Mixed Monarchy*, see Susan Wiseman, "'Adam, the Father of all Flesh': Porno-Political Rhetoric and Political Theory in and After the English Civil War," in *Pamphlet Wars: Prose in the English Revolution*, ed., James Holstun (London: Frank Cass, 1992). Though primarily interested in the relations between political polemic and satiric sexual slander in the Civil War period, Wiseman demonstrates how common it was in patriarchal texts both learned and popular to trace the right of absolute monarchy to Adam's status as absolute father.

18   See Filmer, *Patriarcha*, 10–11.

19   Filmer, "Original of Government," 192.

20   As Weil rightly notes, physiological paternity was not the main ground of Filmer's claim for the father's rule (*Political Passions*, 36), but that it mattered to his position seems evident from his repeated recourse to Adam's single status as generator of his children. One way in which Filmer's opponents, particularly later in the century, sought to undermine his position of fatherly right was to call attention to its most extreme logical implications. Locke, for example, associated Filmer's ideas with the Incas of Peru, who, he said, cannibalized the children they sired from female captives and then ate their mothers, too, when they were past childbearing. See Weil, *Political Passions*, 31ff.

21   In a feminist analysis of the origins of modern political theory, Carole Pate-

man claims that "the patriarchal story is about the procreative power of a father who is complete in himself. His procreative power both gives and nurtures physical life and creates and maintains political right" (*Sexual Contract*, 38). Pateman's is perhaps the most influential of feminist studies on gender and the emergence of modern liberal political theory. Questioning the idea that liberalism was a positive development for women, Pateman argues that liberalism did not so much undermine men's authority over women as transfer it to another register—the private realm of the naturally conceived rather than the politically understood family. Though widely accepted, Pateman's argument has its detractors, too. For example, Schochet, in "Significant Sounds of Silence: the Absence of Women from the Political Thought of Sir Robert Filmer and John Locke (or, 'Why Can't a Woman be More Like a Man?')" in *Women Writers and the Early Modern British Political Tradition*, ed., Hilda Smith (Cambridge: Cambridge University Press, 1998), argues that "Lockean voluntarism . . . opens up the context of 'person' and makes possible political membership and significance beyond the narrow realm of white males" (223). On the changing interplay between discourses of family and state in late Stuart England and particularly in relation to gender, see Rachel Weil, *Political Passions*, whose introduction provides a useful overview of recent trends in scholarship on political modernity and gender. See also Susan Amussen, *An*

*Ordered Society: Class and Gender in Early Modern England* (Oxford: Basil Blackwell, 1998). On the use of the analogy between family and state specifically in the civil war period, see Mary Shanley, "Marriage Contract and Social Contract in Seventeenth-Century Political Thought," *Western Political Quarterly* 32 (1979), and Ann Hughes, "Gender and Politics in Leveller Literature" in *Political Culture and Cultural Politics in Early Modern England*, ed. Susan Amussen and Mark Kishlansky (Manchester: Manchester University Press, 1995).

22  I am using here Pateman's distinction between paternal and masculine right: in her analysis of the transformations of patriarchy in the classical political theories of the seventeenth century, Pateman notes, "Patriarchalism has two dimensions: the paternal (father/son) and the masculine (husband/wife)" (*Sexual Contract*, 37). In this chapter, I construe masculine right in the more general terms of man's right over woman, as opposed to a specifically conjugal right.

23  The two positive contributions for which *De generatione* is famous in the history of medicine are Harvey's identification of the cicatricula (or blastoderm) as the point of origin of the chick in the hen's egg and his reintroduction of epigenesis as the theory governing embryogenesis. See Needham, *History of Embryology*, 133ff.

24  Harvey's fullest explanation of the egg, or "primordium," as he sometimes called it, is as follows: "All Living things do derive their Original (as we have said) from something, which

doth contain in it both the matter and efficient virtue and power; which therefore is that thing, both out of which and by which, whatsoever is born, doth deduce its beginning. And such as Original or Rudiment in Animals (whether they proceed from other Animals which do beget them, or else are spontaneous, and the Issues of Putrefaction) is a certain humour, which is concluded in some certain coat, or shell; namely, a similar body, having life actually in it, or in potentia: and this, in case it be generated within an Animal, is commonly called a Conception: but if it be exposed without, by being born, or else assume its beginning elsewhere, it is called either an Egg or a Worm. But I conceive that both ought alike to be called Primordium, the first Rudiment from which an Animal doth spring; as Plants assume their nativity from the Seed: and all these Primordia are of one kinde, namely Vital" (*DG*, 514–15). A viviparous "conception" is thus to be understood as analogous to an oviparous "egg," that is, a primary something that has vitality, either actually (if fertilized) or potentially.

25  For more detailed accounts of Harvey's understanding of the egg, see Gasking, *Investigations into Generation*, 27–29, and Needham, *History of Embryology*, 133–53.

26  In his 1847 translation of *De generatione*, Robert Willis neatly characterized Harvey's debt not only to Aristotle but to his teacher, Fabricius, as well. Harvey, he says, "begins by putting himself in some sort into the harness of Aristotle, and taking the bit of Fabri-

cius between his teeth; and then, either assuming the ideas of the former as premises, or those of the latter as topics of discussion or dissent, he labours on endeavouring to find Nature in harmony with the Stagyrite, or at variance with the professor of Padua . . . " (William Harvey, *Anatomical Exercises on the Generation of Animals*, in *The Works of William Harvey*, trans. Robert Willis (London: Sydenham Society, 1847), lxx–lxxi. On Harvey's commitment to Aristotelianism generally, see Pagel, *Harvey's Biological Ideas*, and *New Light on Harvey*.

27  Aristotle, *Generation of Animals*, trans., A. Platt, in *The Complete Works of Aristotle*, ed. J. Barnes (Princeton: Princeton University Press, 1984), 729.b.15f.

28  For gender-inflected readings of biological theories, both ancient and modern, as well as for more detailed accounts of Aristotelian and Galenic embryology, see, for example, Flemming, *Medicine and the Making of Roman Women*; Maryanne Cline Horowitz, "The 'Science' of Embryology before the Discovery of the Ovum," in *Connecting Spheres: Women in the Western World: 1500–Present*, ed. Marilyn Boxer and Jean Quataert (New York: Oxford University Press, 1987); Londa Schiebinger, *The Mind Has No Sex?: Women in the Origins of Modern Science* (Cambridge, Mass: Harvard University Press, 1989); and Nancy Tuana, *The Less Noble Sex: Scientific, Religious, and Philosophical Conceptions of Woman's Nature* (Bloomington: Indiana University Press, 1993).

29  Rogers, *Matter of Revolution*, 15.

30  The term *contagion* did not have a pre-

cise medical meaning in the early modern period. It was often associated indiscriminately with *infection* and, like that term, carried with it the idea of pollution and the spread of impurity. Harvey, however, seems to be emphasizing here less the aspect of disease and more the sense of mimetic propagation. In the mid-sixteenth century, Frascastoro had advanced a theory of contagion based on the transmission of airborne seeds, which perhaps Harvey is thinking of here. See Margaret Pelling, "Contagion/Germ Theory/Specificity," in *Companion Encyclopedia of the History of Medicine*, ed., W. F. Bynum and Roy Porter, 2 vols. (London: Routledge, 1993), 1.309–34. Vivian Nutton discusses the history of the concept of contagion in "The Seeds of Disease: an Explanation of Contagion and Infection from the Greeks to the Renaissance," *Medical History* 27 (1983): 1–34.

31  Harvey's understanding of the uterus as analogous to the brain in its ability to conceive bears some relation to the commonplace idea, ancient in origin, that the maternal imagination is able to transmit to the body of the fetus the marks of a woman's fancies, desires, and intentions. Thus, for example, a child's harelip might be explained by noting that the mother looked at a rabbit while having sex. If a woman were having an affair, she might be able to hide the evidence that might otherwise appear in possible progeny by thinking intently of her husband while having sex with her lover. The difference between

these formulations and what Harvey here proposes is twofold: first, Harvey is talking about the initial moment of conception, the first coming-to-be of the organism, rather than its particular characteristics that emerge over the course of gestation; second, and more tellingly, Harvey is not talking about the power of the imagination per se, but the power of the uterus understood through an analogy to the brain. The uterus, like the brain, is able to reproduce something outside it, something foreign to it. The uterus is a medium of *re-production*, not itself a creator. Against the common understanding of the power of the maternal imagination to form things like itself, Harvey's analogy works to make the uterus something that forms things like the father. On the maternal imagination from the Renaissance through the Enlightenment, see part one in Marie-Hélène Huet, *Monstrous Imagination* (Cambridge, Mass.: Harvard University Press, 1993). On the maternal imagination specifically as it is discussed in a healthcare manual often reprinted in the late seventeenth and eighteenth centuries, see Mary Fissell, "'Hairy Women and Naked Truths.'"

32  On Jonas, see chapter 3, above.

33  Thomas Hobbes, *Leviathan*, ed. C. B. Macpherson (Harmondsworth, Middlesex: Penguin Books, 1968), 254. Although *Leviathan* was first published in 1651, similar comments appear in earlier versions of Hobbes's political theory, as, for example, in *The Citizen*, first published in 1642: "In the state of nature, every woman that bears chil-

dren, becomes both a *mother* and a *lord*"; see Thomas Hobbes, *Man and Citizen*, ed. Bernard Gert (Gloucester, Mass.: Peter Smith, 1978), 213.

34 Christine Di Stefano, *Configurations of Masculinity: A Feminist Perspective on Modern Political Theory* (Ithaca: Cornell University Press, 1991), 85.

35 Hobbes, *Man and Citizen*, 205. See Di Stefano, *Configurations of Masculinity*, 83ff., for a detailed analysis of Hobbes's mushroom image. See also Carole Pateman, "'God Hath Ordained to Man a Helper': Hobbes, Patriarchy and Conjugal Right," in *Feminist Interpretations and Political Theory*, ed. Mary Lyndon Shanley and Carole Pateman (Cambridge: Polity Press, 1990), 53–73.

36 Di Stefano, *Configurations of Masculinity*, 82–83.

37 Carole Pateman, *The Disorder of Women: Democracy, Feminism, and Political Theory* (Stanford: Stanford University Press, 1989), 37.

38 Pateman, "God Hath Ordained," 54–56.

39 Of the many treatments of this image, see, for example, Evelyn Fox Keller, "Baconian Science: A Hermaphroditic Birth," *Philosophical Forum* 11 (1980): 299–308.

40 For an analysis of anatomical illustrations in Renaissance texts in which the dissected subjects appear willingly and even erotically to display themselves before the anatomist's knife, see Jonathan Sawday, "The Fate of Marsyas: Dissecting the Renaissance Body," in *Renaissance Bodies: The Human Figure in English Culture c. 1540–1660*, ed. Lucy Gent and Nigel Llewellyn (London: Reaktion, 1990).

## 5 / Embryonic Individuals: Mechanism, Embryology, and Modern Man

1 *Philosophical Transactions of the Royal Society*, 1672, vol. 7, no. 18: 4021 (hereafter cited as *PT*).

2 Ibid., 4021.

3 Ibid., 4022.

4 Ibid.

5 Jacques Roger's monumental history of eighteenth-century "sciences of life" in France, *Les sciences de la vie*, situates debates about embryogeny in the context of contemporary concerns about epistemology and philosophical questions about the origin of animal form. Shirley Roe's book on the Haller-Wolff debates (*Matter, Life, and Generation* [1981]) attempts to demonstrate the indebtedness of questions about generation to a priori questions about methodology and philosophy of nature. See also Gasking, *Investigations into Generation*; Helmut Muller-Sievers, *Self-Generation: Biology, Philosophy, and Literature around 1800* (Stanford: Stanford University Press, 1997); and Clara Pinto-Carreia, *The Ovary of Eve: Egg and Sperm and Preformation* (Chicago: University of Chicago Press, 1997).

6 René Descartes, *Discourse of the Method of Properly Conducting One's Reason and of Seeking the Truth in the Sciences*, 1637, trans. F. E. Sutcliffe (Harmondsworth: Penguin Books, 1968), 73; Robert Boyle, *The Usefulness of Experimental Philosophy*, in *The Works of the Honourable Robert Boyle*, ed. Thomas Birch, 6 vols. (Hildesheim: Olms, 1965–1966), 2.75–76. On the rise of mechanism in English

physiology generally, see Theodore Brown, *The Mechanical Philosophy and the "Animal Oeconomy"* (New York: Arno Press, 1981).

7   Francis Bacon, *Francis Bacon: A Selection of his Works*, ed. Sidney Warhaft (Indianapolis: Bobbs-Merrill Educational Publishing, 1965), 330.

8   *The Compact Edition of the Oxford English Dictionary* (Oxford: Oxford University Press, 1971), 1.1756 and 1687.

9   Cited in the *OED*, 1.1756. As applied to persons, the word was also associated with the laboring class. See Patricia Parker, "Rude Mechanicals," in *Subject and Object in Renaissance Culture*, eds., Margreta de Grazia, Maureen Quilligan, and Peter Stallybrass (Cambridge: Cambridge University Press, 1996), 43.

10  Margreta de Grazia, Maureen Quilligan, and Peter Stallybrass, the editors of *Subjects and Objects in Renaissance Culture* (Cambridge: Cambridge University Press, 1996), ask after the status of the object "in the period that has from its inception been identified with the emergence of the subject." What happens, they wonder, "once the object is brought into view? What new configurations will emerge when subject and object are kept in relation?" (2). My effort here is to take up one aspect of their question: what happens, I want to ask, when the subject is *itself* an object—both as the thing that is studied and, perhaps, as no more than a thing itself? What happens when a dissected clot of blood is an infant and an engine?

11  Sawday, *Body Emblazoned*, 113.

12  Ibid., 113–14.

13  Ibid., 115. For a reading of these illus-

trations that takes account of their gender implications, see Valerie Traub, "Gendering Mortality in Early Modern Anatomies," in *Feminist Readings of Early Modern Culture: Emerging Subjects*, ed. Valerie Traub, M. Lindsay Kaplan, and Dympna Callaghan (Cambridge: Cambridge University Press, 1996).

14  John M. Riddle, *Contraception and Abortion from the Ancient World to the Renaissance* (Cambridge, Mass.: Harvard University Press, 1992), 158.

15  Ibid., 112.

16  Ibid., 18.

17  Edward Coke, *The Third Part of the Institutes of the Laws of England* (London, 1644), 50, as quoted in Angus McLaren, *Reproductive Rituals: The Perception of Fertility in England from the Sixteenth to the Nineteenth Century* (London: Methuen, 1984), 121.

18  McLaren defines "misprison" as a noncapital common-law offence such as bribing a witness or attacking a judge. Chapter 5 of *Reproductive Rituals* provides a useful overview of the medical, legal, and religious arguments preceding the 1803 law that made abortion a statutory offence.

19  These examples and many others like them are to be found in McLaren, *Reproductive Rituals*, 103.

20  Ibid., 108.

21  Guillemeau, *Childbirth*, 69–70; Maubray, *The Female Physician* (London: Holland, 1724), 24–28; both cited in McLaren, *Reproductive Rituals*, 108.

22  William Sermon, *The Ladies Companion, or, The English Midwife* (London: E. Thomas, 1671), 19.

23 Ibid., 16; Sharp, *Midwives Book*, 82. On the indeterminacy of early pregnancy, particularly seen through the writings of Englishwomen preserved in English Record Offices, see Laura Gowing, *Common Bodies: Women, Touch and Power in Seventeenth-Century England* (New Haven: Yale University Press, 2003), 113–22.

24 See, for example, Sermon, who calls pregnancy "the greatest disease that can afflict women," *Ladies Companion*, B1v. On the association of the pregnant body with disease, especially in the eighteenth century, see Barbara Duden, *The Woman Beneath the Skin: A Doctor's Patients in Eighteenth-Century Germany*, trans. Thomas Dunlap (Cambridge, Mass.: Harvard University Press, 1991).

25 Sermon, *Ladies Companion*, 31.

26 McLaren, *Reproductive Rituals*, 46.

27 Sharp, *Midwives Book*, 81–83.

28 Aristotle (pseudonym), *Aristotle's Master-piece, or, The Secrets of Generation* (London: Printed for W. B., 1694), 46. For a historical survey of English-language treatises dealing with sexual knowledge after the middle of the seventeenth century, see Porter and Hall, eds., *The Facts of Life*.

29 Sermon distinguishes between the stirring of a child (later in gestation) and the motion of a mole, which might easily be mistaken for the same thing, by explaining that the latter "proceeds from the expulsive faculty of the mother" rather than from the desire of a living child seeking air. One way to tell the difference is to see if, when the woman lies on her side, the weight "fall[s] like a bowl"; if it does,

it is probably a mole. Sermon, *Ladies Companion*, 35.

30 The dissociation between the fetus and the mother's body becomes especially evident when these images are compared with the famous illustrations of the gravid uterus from the eighteenth century done by William Hunter and William Smellie. See Ludmilla Jordanova, "Gender, Generation, and Science: William Hunter's Obstetrical Atlas," in *William Hunter and the Eighteenth-Century Medical World*, ed. W. F. Bynum and Roy Porter (Cambridge: Cambridge University Press, 1985). Also see Andrea Henderson, "Doll-Machines and Butcher-Shop Meat: Models of Childbirth in the Early Stages of Industrial Capitalism," *Genders* 12 (Winter, 1991): 100–119 on how differences in the representation of the maternal body in Smellie's and Hunter's texts suggest a transition in the understanding of the mother's role in reproduction.

31 The earliest appear in a thirteenth-century gynecological manuscript by Muscio, and various versions subsequently appear in many of the midwifery manuals of the early modern period, most popularly in *The Byrth of Mankynde*, see plate 4 on page 77. For a survey of gynecological images, see Harold Speert, *Iconographia Gyniatrica: A Pictorial History of Gynecology and Obstetrics* (Philadelphia: F. A. Davis, 1973). See Newman, *Fetal Positions*, on these specific images, discussed below.

32 Newman, *Fetal Positions*, 26. See also p. 82: "The woman-as-reproductive-body, as mother, cannot be allowed to encroach upon or trouble the identifi-

catory relay between observing subject and fetal body."

33 Laura Gowing rightly points out that some midwifery texts, such as Jane Sharp's *Midwives Book* (121), include images drawn from anatomy illustrations that show the fetus curled within the revealed uterus of a whole-bodied mother. She further notes that these images are embedded in texts that "describe in detail the dependency of the foetus on the mother: her diet, her behaviour, her temperament" (*Common Bodies*, 125). This, she argues, has the effect of undermining the presumed fetal autonomy urged by the fetus-in-womb images and promotes instead the worry that women need reminding how much the welfare of their progeny depends on their behavior (126). I would add, though, that Sharp's inclusion of the mother's body in the image still deals with questions relating to the status of a *mature* fetus, not the status of an embryo.

34 Through much of the sixteenth century, research efforts were largely (though not exclusively) devoted to the description of fetal anatomy, rather than to the systematic observation of the course of development of an animal. Though Aldrovandi, for example, did daily dissect twenty-two eggs a hen was incubating, his description of the results takes up only two pages of a three-volume work on ornithology. And Aldrovandi's interest in charting the daily changes of a chick's embryo was, along with the work of Coiter, the exception rather than the rule in the course of sixteenth-century research.

See Adelman, *Malpighi and the Evolution of Embryology*, 2.753ff. For the history of embryological research from the sixteenth through the eighteenth centuries, see F. J. Cole, *Early Theories of Sexual Generation* (Oxford: Clarendon Press, 1930); Roger, *Les sciences*; Gasking, *Investigations into Generation*; Needham, *History of Embryology*; Roe, *Matter, Life, Generation*.

35 Most, though not all, of the theories of the time were not purely vitalist or mechanistic, but combined aspects of both, though in widely varying degrees. So, for example, Kerckring's theory, though essentially mechanistic, did admit an element of vitalism to explain conception itself; it held that the spiritual force of the semen fecundates the ovum in the female testicle, thereby propelling it through the Fallopian tubes into the matrix where it almost immediately emerges as a "child."

36 On the ambiguity of these classificatory terms even in modern scholarship on embryology, see Frederick Churchill, "The History of Embryology as Intellectual History," *Journal of the History of Biology* 3.1 (Spring, 1970): 155–81, and Peter Bowler, "Preformation and Preexistence in the Seventeenth Century: A Brief Analysis," *Journal of the History of Biology* 4.2 (Fall, 1971): 221–44.

37 See Daniel Fouke, "Mechanical and 'Organical' Models in Seventeenth-Century Explanations of Biological Reproduction," *Science in Context* 3.2 (Autumn, 1989): 366–81.

38 Kenelm Digby, *Two Treatises* (Paris: Gilles Blaizot, 1644), 215 (hereafter cited as *TT*). Digby's discussion of

nutrition is not original to him but derives from the pre-Socratic philosopher, Anaxagoras.

39  F. J. Cole terms Digby's theory "speculative epigenesis," since it is so little based on his empirical findings (*Early Theories of Sexual Generation*, 157), and Adelmann says, "certainly it cannot be said that [Digby's] theory of generation bears any direct relation to this own experience with the developing chick" (*Malpighi and the Evolution of Embryology*, 770).

40  George Garden represented a familiar sentiment when he reminded readers "how wretchedly Descartes came off in this matter" of attempting a mechanical explanation for epigenetic generation. See *Philosophical Transactions*, 1691, no. 192:477.

41  Quoted in Roe, *Matter, Life, and Generation*, 1. On the failure of mechanical epigenesis, see A. J. Pyle, "Animal Generation and the Mechanical Philosophy: Some Light on the Role of Biology in the Scientific Revolution," *History and Philosophy of the Life Sciences* 9 (1987): 225–54, and Fouke, "Mechanical and 'Organical.'"

42  Since Harvey began his research on generation in the 1630s, over a decade before Digby's theory was published, his work was not a response to Digby per se; but when Harvey chose to publish his own material in 1651, his ideas entered an ongoing debate about the explanatory sufficiency of vitalism and mechanism, and so his work, though not particularly a response to Digby, is in part a response to the difficulties that mechanical explanation posed.

43  Nathaniel Highmore, *The History of Generation* (London: John Martin, 1651), 86 (hereafter cited as *HG*).

44  The soul not only ensures that the new individuum is of the same species as its parents; it also determines its minute structures: "The principles . . . of these living births, arise . . . from some selected Atoms by the testicles of both [male and female], thrown into the Matrix of the Female. Where being united & mixt by the fermenting heat of the Womb: the several Atomes fall to their respective places: the soul playing the skilful Workman, (not laying brick where should be morter) reposing every Atome in his proper place, that very same which it should have held in the body, from when it was separated" (*HG*, 86).

45  Again, as in chapter 4, this alignment between the physiological and the political occurs despite the fact that Harvey was an ardent Royalist. The argument is not that Harvey *intentionally* promoted this view; rather that the physiological rhetoric nonetheless participates in a larger cultural pattern that assumes it.

46  Claude Perrault, for example, in his "La Mechanique des animaux" (1680), objected to mechanical epigenesis on precisely these theological grounds: "I do not know if one can comprehend how a work of this quality would be the effect of the ordinary forces of nature . . . for I find finally that it is scarcely more inconceivable . . . that the world has been able to form itself from matter out of chaos, than an ant can form another from the homogeneous substance of the semen from

which it is believed to be engendered." Quoted in Roe, *Matter, Life, and Generation*, 8. See also Pyle, "Animal Generation and Mechanical Philosophy."

47   Gasking, *Investigations into Generation*, 42; Pyle, "Animal Generation and Mechanical Philosophy." Metamorphosis and preformation differ mostly in the points at which they assert the existence of heterogeneity: in metamorphosis it is the conception that is heterogeneous; in preformation the egg or the animalcule is. Neither theory, however, addresses how complexity and life actually arise.

48   Jane Oppenheimer, *History of Embryology* (see esp. 134–35), has suggested that it is no coincidence that epigenesis (the theory favored by Digby and Harvey) was eventually accepted in the late eighteenth century, at a time when revolution and the question of political obligation were once again raised.

49   Croone gave his manuscript on the development of the chick in the egg to the Royal Society in March, 1671; in 1672, an abstract of the paper was published in *Philosophical Transactions*. In 1757, the journal published the entire paper. See F. J. Cole, "Dr. William Croone On Generation" [1946], in *Studies and Essays in the History of Science and Learning*, ed. M. F. Ashley Montagu (New York: Arno Press, 1975), 115–35. This article includes Cole's translation of Croone's complete Latin text. My citations are to this translation, hereafter cited in text as *OG*.

50   Cole, "Croone on Generation," 116.

51   Pre-existence theories such as *emboitement* are the most mechanical of all,

since they restrict all sense of generation to the original divine creation of the universe. But pre-existence did not really take hold until the eighteenth century, though some, like Malebranche, supported it earlier, and others, like Swammerdam, speculated about it. Swammerdam said he considered it very probable "that in the whole course of things there is no generation that can be properly so called, nor can anything else be observed, than the continuation as it were of generation already performed." Quoted in Abraham Schierbeek, *Jan Swammerdam, 12 February 1637–17 February 1680: His Life and Works* (Amsterdam: Swets Zeitlinger, 1967), 115.

52   *Philosophical Transactions*, 1670, no. 64:2079–80.

53   Fouke, "Mechanical and 'Organical,'" 373–75.

54   *Philosophical Transactions*, 1670, no. 64:2079.

55   On Swammerdam's indebtedness to vitalism, see Fouke, "Mechanical and 'Organical,'" 373.

56   *Philosophical Transactions*, 1683, no. 147: 187.

57   Tuana, *The Less Noble Sex*, 150, and Horowitz, "The 'Science' of Embryology."

58   De Graff actually discovered the ovarian follicles but these were initially taken to be eggs. See Needham, *History of Embryology*, 163.

59   Edward Ruestow, "Leeuwenhoek's Perception of the Spermatozoa," *Journal of the History of Biology*, 6.2 (1983): 196.

60   Thus, according to Shirley Roe, the rise of preformationist theories in the late seventeenth century was a

response to "a series of philosophical problems posed by the application of mechanical explanation to embryology," including the function of God in the process of generation. Roe, *Matter, Life, and Generation*, 8.

61 Ralph Cudworth, *The True Intellectual System of the Universe* (1678; repr., Stuttgart-Bad Cannstatt: Friedrich Frommann Verlag, 1964), 761.

62 Humphrey Ditton, *The New Law of Fluids* (London, 1714), 23–24; quoted in Yolton, *Thinking Matter*, 43.

63 Henderson, "Doll-Machines and Butcher-Shop Meat."

64 For a brief biographical sketch of Garden and for a reading of his paper, particularly in the context of his religious and theological commitments, see Anita Guerrini, "The Burden of Procreation: Women and Preformation in the Works of George Garden and George Cheyne," in *Science and Medicine in the Scottish Enlightenment*, ed. Charles W. J. Withers and Paul Woods (East Linton: Tuckwell Press, 2002). For more on Garden's career, see Anita Guerrini, *Obesity and Depression in the Enlightenment: The Life and Times of George Cheyne* (Norman, OK: University of Oklahoma Press, 2000), 13–15.

65 *Philosophical Transactions*, 1691, no. 192: 474.

66 Ibid.:480.

67 *Philosophical Transactions*, 1682, no. 145: 76.

68 *Philosophical Transactions*, 1685, no. 174: 1133.

69 The figures appeared in *Philosophical Transactions* along with Leeuwenhoeck's refutation of Dalenpatius's

claim that he had seen the legs, breast, arms, and head of an animalcule (1699, no. 255, interleaved before page 269).

## 6 / The Masculine Subject of Touch: Case Histories from the Birthing Room

1 Edmund Chapman, *Essay on the Improvement of Midwifery* (London: A. Blackwell, 1733), 89 (hereafter cited as *IM*).

2 Lisa Cody's *Birthing the Nation* examines the alignment of men's new assumption of authority in childbirth with questions of individual and corporate identity in the eighteenth century. Her book brings an important and sophisticated new perspective to this well-rehearsed story. See my introduction here, notes 5 and 6.

3 James H. Aveling, *English Midwives: Their History and Prospects* (1872; repr., London: Hugh K. Elliott, 1967) typifies this style. He has this to say about four men who practiced midwifery in the seventeenth century: William Harvey, Peter Chamberlen, William Sermon, and Percival Willughby were, he asserts, "men of high social and medical position. Had they considered the study and practice of midwifery beneath their dignity, how disastrous would it have been to English mothers, and who can say how much longer the dark ages of midwifery would have continued in this country" (46). This perspective persists in works as recent as Edward Shorter, *Women's Bodies: A Social History of Women's Encounter with Health,*

*Ill-Health and Medicine* (New Brunswick, N.J.: Transaction Publications, 1991).

4 Typical of this mode is Barbara Ehrenreich and Deirdre English, *Witches, Midwives and Nurses* (Old Westbury, N.Y.: Feminist Press, 1973). For brief summaries of the extensive scholarship, see the chapter on "Doctors and Women" in Dorothy Porter and Roy Porter, *Patient's Progress: Doctors and Doctoring in Eighteenth-Century England* (Stanford: Stanford University Press, 1989) and the introduction in Doreen Evenden, *The Midwives of Seventeenth-Century London* (Cambridge: Cambridge University Press, 2000).

5 Cody, "Politics of Reproduction: From Midwives' Alternative Pubic Sphere to the Public Spectacle of Man Midwifery," *Eighteenth-Century Studies* 32.4 (1999): 478.

6 Adrian Wilson, *The Making of Man-Midwifery: Childbirth in England, 1660–1770* (Cambridge, Mass.: Harvard University Press, 1995), esp. chapter 14.

7 Ibid., 181.

8 Evenden, *Midwives of Seventeenth-Century London*, 175.

9 Sharp, *Midwives Book*, 11–12. See also Eve Keller, "Mrs. Jane Sharp: Midwifery and the Critique of Medical Knowledge."

10 Sarah Stone, *A Complete Practice of Midwifery* (London: T. Cooper, 1737), vii; x (hereafter cited as *CPM*). On Stone, see Isobel Grundy, "Sarah Stone: Englightenment Midwife," in *Medicine and the Enlightenment*, ed. Roy Porter (Amsterdam: Rodopi, 1994), which analyzes Stone's use of heroic romance and scriptural narrative conventions to portray herself as an Enlightenment hero.

11 On the limited exposure of most male practitioners to normal deliveries, see Wilson, *Man-Midwifery*, 47–59. This changed dramatically only after the mid-eighteenth century.

12 Willughby, *Observations in Midwifery*, introduction by John L. Thornton (1863; repr., Wakefield: S.R. Publishers, 1972), 88 (hereafter cited as *OM*). Willughby's work was not published until the nineteenth century but it probably circulated in manuscript to some extent during Willughby's lifetime, and the transcripts were likely made after his death. See Thornton's introduction, x–xiii.

13 For a detailed description of the role of male practitioners in the birthing room through the early eighteenth century, see Wilson, *Man-Midwifery*, 47–59.

14 Sharp, *Midwives Book*, 148–49.

15 Ibid., 149.

16 Elliptical information on the use of surgeon's instruments was standard in some midwifery books. *The Byrth of Mankynde*, for example, included it, though Guillemeau's *Child-birth, or, The Happy Deliuerie of Vvomen* (1612) did not. Much of Sharp's manual is derived from previously published material (such as Culpeper's *Directory for Midwives*), and this sketch of using surgical instruments is not original to her; still, in the context of her general effort to counter the intrusion of surgeons into the birthing room, Sharp's promotion of midwives using surgical instruments reads as a defense of a midwife's professional preserve.

17 Helen King, "'As if None Understood the Art that Cannot Understand Greek': The Education of Midwives

in Seventeenth-Century England," in *The History of Medical Education in Britain*, ed. Vivian Nutton and Roy Porter (Amsterdam: Rodopi, 1995), 189.

18  *A Directory for Midwives*, for example, includes prefaces by both Culpeper and his wife that testify to the authenticity of the many books he wrote and translated.

19  Roy Porter, "The Rise of Physical Examination," in *Medicine and the Five Senses*, ed. W. F. Bynum and Roy Porter (Cambridge: Cambridge University Press, 1993), 182.

20  Ibid., 183.

21  Ibid.

22  Another reason that physical examination was not deemed necessary for accurate diagnosis is that, within the context of humoral medicine, disease was understood to be caused by an imbalance of an individual's idiosyncratic humoral complexion, which itself was best determined by considering a person's complete lifestyle, as we saw in chapter 1. See also Beier, *Sufferers and Healers*, 31ff.

23  On the permeability of boundaries between learned and popular medicine, see Wear, "Popularization of Medicine in Early Modern England" (see p. 19 for this list of kinds of practitioners).

24  On the absence of physical contact between physician and patient, see S. J. Reiser, *Medicine and the Reign of Technology* (Cambridge: Cambridge University Press, 1978), 5–6, and Malcolm Nicolson, "The Art of Diagnosis: Medicine and the Five Senses," in *Companion Encyclopedia of the History of Medicine*, ed. W. F. Bynum and Roy

Porter (London: Routledge, 1993), 2.801–25. Also see Porter, "Rise of Physical Examination," 180.

25  W. F. Bynum, "Health, Disease and Medical Care," in *The Ferment of Knowledge: Studies in the Historiography of Eighteenth-Century Science*, ed. G. Rousseau and R. Porter (Cambridge: Cambridge University Press, 1980), 211.

26  John Symcotts, *A Seventeenth-Century Doctor and His Patients: John Symcotts, 1592?–1662*, ed. F. N. L. Poynter and W. J. Bishop. Publications of the Bedfordshire Historical Record Society 31 (Streatley: Bedfordshire Publication Society, 1951), 14 (hereafter cited as *JS*).

27  Henry van Deventer, *The Art of Midwifery Improv'd*, trans. Robert Samber (London: E. Curll, J. Pemberton, and W. Taylor, 1716), A3v (hereafter cited as *AMI*).

28  Adrian Wilson, "Participant versus Patient: Seventeenth-Century Childbirth from the Mother's Point of View," in *Patients and Practitioners: Lay Perceptions of Medicine in Pre-Industrial Society*, ed. Roy Porter (Cambridge: Cambridge University Press, 1986), 129–44. See also chapter 3 here.

29  Although podalic version was known in ancient times, it was a technique apparently lost to the West until the sixteenth century, when Ambroise Paré reintroduced it into medical texts, but even after that, it only slowly entered vernacular medical literature.

30  On the association of male midwifery and obscenity, especially in the later eighteenth century, see Roy Porter, "A Touch of Danger: The Man-Midwife as Sexual Predator," in *Sexual Under-*

*worlds of the Enlightenment*, ed. G. S. Rousseau and Roy Porter (Manchester: Manchester University Press, 1987), 206–32.

31  On Willughby's and his daughter's practice, see Adrian Wilson, "A Memorial of Eleanor Willughby, a Seventeenth-Century Midwife," in *Women, Science and Medicine, 1500–1700*, ed. Lynette Hunter and Sarah Hutton (Phoenix Mill: Sutton Publishing, 1997), 128–78. For more details about the extant manuscripts and their publication, also see John L. Thornton's introduction to the 1972 facsimile reprint of Willughby's *Observations*.

32  On Deventer's technical innovations see Wilson, *Making of Man-Midwifery*, 79–85 and H. L. Houtzager, "Hendrik van Deventer," in *European Journal of Obstetrics, Gynaecology and Reproductive Biology* 21 (1986): 263–70. The 1716 English text is a translation of a 1701 Latin translation of the 1701 Dutch original.

33  Deventer was the first to indicate the significance of the size and shape of the pelvis to successful birth outcomes. See Wilson, *Making of Man-Midwifery*, 79.

34  Although not precisely a collection of case histories, Deventer's treatise is an argument for the importance of touch and a fairly explicit and detailed instruction manual for how and when to perform it. Without recording individual cases, it details precisely what he does in any given circumstance.

35  See also Deventer's detailed instructions on how to give a clyster, or enema, which includes the advice, "that the buttocks being separated with the Fingers of one Hand, distending the Anus, the Pipe is gently to be put in with the other, about a Fingers Length . . . " (*AMI*, 108). Instructions as specific as this are quite rare in the contemporary literature.

36  William Giffard, *Cases in Midwifery*, ed. Edward Hody, MD (London: B. Motte and T. Wotton, 1734), 47–49 (hereafter cited as *CM*).

37  For women's responses in the eighteenth century to the rise of male midwifery, see Elizabeth Nihell, *A Treatise on the Art of Midwifery* (London: A. Morely, 1760), and Martha Mears, *The Pupil of Nature* (London: L. Lickfield, 1797). On the accusation that male midwifery was a lecher's sport, see Porter, "Touch of Danger: The Man-Midwife as Sexual Predator."

## Epilogue

1  A similar bill was introduced in the House of Representatives by Chris Smith (R-New Jersey) (HR.356).

2  Joseph A. D'Agostino, "The Next Legislative Battle: Unborn Child Pain Awareness Act," *PRI Briefing* 7.4 (28 January, 2005), available at lifeissue.net/writers/mos/mos_37pain.html.

3  Mitchell, *Me++: The Cyborg Self and the Networked City* (Cambridge, Mass.: MIT Press, 2003), 62.

4  Ibid., 8.

5  Ibid., 22.

# BIBLIOGRAPHY

Adelmann, Howard. *Marcello Malpighi and the Evolution of Embryology*. Ithaca: Cornell University Press, 1966.

Altman, Meryl, and Keith Nightenhelser. "*Making Sex*: Review." *Postmodern Culture* 2, no. 3 (May 1992): http://muse.jhu.edu.avoserv.library.fordham.edu/journals/postmodern_culture/v002/2.3r_altman.html.

Amussen, Susan. *An Ordered Society: Class and Gender in Early Modern England*. Oxford: Basil Blackwell, 1998.

Aristotle. *Generation of Animals: The Revised Oxford Translation*. Translated by A. Platt. In *The Complete Works of Aristotle*, edited by J. Barnes. Princeton: Princeton University Press, 1984.

Aristotle (pseudonym). *Aristotle's Masterpiece, or, The Secrets of Generation*. London: Printed for W. B., 1694.

Aveling, James. *English Midwives: Their History and Prospects*. 1872. Reprint, London: Hugh K. Elliott, 1967.

Bacon, Francis. *Francis Bacon: A Selection of his Works*. Edited by Sidney Warhaft. Indianapolis: Bobbs-Merrill Educational Publishing, 1965.

Ballantyne, J. W. "The Byrth of Mankynde: Its Author and Editions." *Journal of Obstetrics and Gynaecology of the British Empire* 10, no. 4 (1906): 297–326.

———. "The Byrth of Mankynde: Its Contents." *Journal of Obstetrics and Gynaecology of the British Empire* 12, no. 3 (1907): 175–94 and 12, no. 4 (1907): 255–74.

Banister, John. *The Historie of Man*. London, John Daye, 1578.

Barkan, Leonard. *Nature's Work of Art: The Human Body as Image of the World*. New Haven: Yale University Press, 1975.

Beier, Lucinda McCray. *Sufferers and Healers: The Experience of Illness in Seventeenth-Century England*. London: Routledge, 1987.

Belsey, Catherine. *The Subject of Tragedy: Identity and Difference in Renaissance Drama*. London: Methuen, 1985.

Blakeslee, Sandra. "When the Brain Says, 'Don't Get Too Close.'" *New York Times* July 13, 2004, F2.

Bowler, Peter. "Preformation and Pre-existence in the Seventeenth Century: A Brief Analysis." *Journal of the History of Biology* 4, no. 2 (Fall 1971): 221–44.

Boyle, Robert. *The Usefulness of Experimental Philosophy*. Vol. 2 of *The Works of the Honourable Robert Boyle*. Edited by Thomas Birch. Hildesheim: Olms, 1965–1966.

Boss, Jeffrey. "The Seventeenth-Century Transformation of the Hysteric Affection, and Sydenham's Baconian Medicine." *Psychological Medicine* 9 (1979): 221–34.

Brooks, Rodney Allen. *Flesh and Machines: How Robots Will Change Us*. New York: Pantheon Books, 2002.

Brown, Theodore. *The Mechanical Philosophy and the "Animal Oeconomy."* New York: Arno Press, 1981.

Burckhardt, Jacob. *The Civilization of the Renaissance in Italy,* 1859. Oxford: Phaidon, 1981.

Bynum, W. F. "Health, Disease and Medical Care." In *The Ferment of Knowledge: Studies in the Historiography of Eighteenth-Century Science,* edited by G. S. Rousseau and R. Porter. Cambridge: Cambridge University Press, 1980.

Cadden, Joan. *Meanings of Sex Difference in the Middle Ages: Medicine, Science, and Culture.* Cambridge: Cambridge University Press, 1993.

Cantor, David, ed. *Reinventing Hippocrates.* Aldershot: Ashgate, 2002.

Chapman, Edmund. *Essay on the Improvement of Midwifery.* London: A. Blackwell, 1733.

Charleton, Walter. *Natural History of Nutrition, Life, and Voluntary Motion.* London: Henry Herringman, 1659.

Churchill, Frederick. "The History of Embryology as Intellectual History." *Journal of the History of Biology* 3, no. 1 (Spring, 1970): 155–81.

Churchland, Patricia Smith. *Brain-Wise: Studies in Neurophilosophy.* Cambridge, Mass.: MIT Press, 2002.

———.*Neurophilosophy: Towards a Unified Understanding of the Mind-Brain.* Cambridge, Mass.: MIT Press, 1986.

Churchland, Paul M. *Matter and Consciousness: A Contemporary Introduction to the Philosophy of Mind.* rev. ed. Cambridge, Mass.: MIT Press, 1988.

Clark, Andy. *Natural-Born Cyborgs: Minds, Technologies, and the Future of Human Intelligence.* New York: Oxford University Press, 2003.

Clark, George N. *A History of the Royal College of Physicians of London.* 2 vols. Oxford: Clarendon Press, 1964–1966.

Cody, Lisa Forman. *Birthing the Nation: Sex, Science, and the Conception of Eighteenth-Century Britons.* Oxford: Oxford University Press, 2005.

———. "Politics of Reproduction: From Midwives' Alternative Public Sphere to the Public Spectacle of Man Midwifery." *Eighteenth-Century Studies* 32, no.4 (1999): 477–95.

Cohen, I. Bernard. "Harrington and Harvey: A Theory of the State Based on the New Physiology." *Journal of the History of Ideas* 55 (1994): 187–210.

Cohen, Robert S., and Thomas Schnelle, eds. *Cognition and Fact: Materials on Ludwik Fleck.* Dordrecht: D. Reidel Publishing Company, 1986.

Cole, F. J. "Dr. William Croone On Generation." In *Studies and Essays in the History of Science and Learning,* edited by M. F. Ashley Montagu. 1946. Reprint, New York: Arno Press, 1975.

———. *Early Theories of Sexual Generation.* Oxford: Clarendon Press, 1930..

Cook, Harold. *The Decline of the Old Medical Regime in Stuart London.* Ithaca: Cornell University Press, 1986.

Crawford, Patricia. "Attitudes to Menstruation in Seventeenth-century England." *Past and Present* 91 (1981): 47–73.

———. "The Construction and Experience of Maternity in Seventeenth-Century England." In *Women as Mothers in Pre-Industrial England: Essays in Memory of Dorothy McLaren,* edited by Valerie Fildes. London: Routledge, 1990.

Cressy, David. *Birth, Marriage, and Death: Ritual, Religion, and the Life-Cycle in*

*Tudor and Stuart England*. Oxford: Oxford University Press, 1997.

Crooke, Helkiah. *Microcosmographia: A Description of the Body of Man*. London: William Jaggard, 1615.

Cudworth, Ralph. *The True Intellectual System of the Universe*. 1678. Reprint, Stuttgart-Bad Cannstatt: Friedrich Frommann Verlag, 1964.

Culpeper, Nicholas. *Culpeper's School of Physic*. London: N. Brook, 1659.

———. *A Directory for Midwives, or A Guide for Women*. 2nd ed. London: Peter Cole, 1656.

———. *A Physicall Directory, or, A Translation of the London Dispensatory*. London: Peter Cole, 1649.

———, Abdiah Cole, and William Rowland, trans. *The Practice of Physicke*, by Lazarus Riverius. London: George Sawbridge, 1678.

Cunningham, A., and O. Grell, eds. *Religio Medici: Medicine and Religion in Seventeenth-Century England*. London: Scolar Press, 1996.

Damasio, Antonio R. *The Feeling of What Happens: Body and Emotion in the Making of Consciousness*. New York: Harcourt Brace, 1999.

de Grazia, Margreta, Maureen Quilligan, and Peter Stallybrass, eds. *Subject and Object in Renaissance Culture*. Cambridge: Cambridge University Press, 1996.

Descartes, Rene. *Discourse on the Method of Properly Conducting One's Reason and of Seeking the Truth in the Sciences*. 1637. Translated by F. E. Sutcliffe. Harmondsworth: Penguin Books, 1968.

Digby, Kenelm. *Two Treatises*. Paris: Gilles Blaizot, 1644.

Di Stefano, Christine. *Configurations of Masculinity: A Feminist Perspective on Modern Political Theory*. Ithaca: Cornell University Press, 1991.

Duden, Barbara. *The Woman Beneath the Skin: A Doctor's Patients in Eighteenth-Century Germany*. Translated by Thomas Dunlap. Cambridge, Mass.: Harvard University Press, 1991.

Durling, R. J. "A Chronological Census of Renaissance Editions and Translations of Galen." *Journal of the Warburg and Cortauld Institute* 24 (1961): 230–305.

Eccles, Audrey. *Obstetrics and Gynaecology in Tudor and Stuart England*. Kent, Ohio: Kent State University Press, 1982.

Edelman, Gerald M. *Bright Air, Brilliant Fire: On the Matter of Mind*. New York: Basic Books, 1992.

———, and Giulio Tononi. *A Universe of Consciousness: How Matter Becomes Imagination*. New York: Basic Books, 2000.

Ehrenreich, Barbara, and Deirdre English. *Witches, Midwives and Nurses*. Old Westbury, NY: Feminist Press, 1973.

Elyot, Thomas. *The Castel of Health*. 1541 [1536]. Facsimile edition. New York: Scholar's Facsimiles, 1936.

Erickson, Robert. "The Books of Generation: Some Observations on the Style of the English Midwife Books, 1671–1764." In *Sexuality in Eighteenth-Century Britain*, edited by Paul-Gabriel Boucé. Manchester: Manchester University Press, 1982.

Evenden, Doreen. *The Midwives of Seventeenth-Century London*. Cambridge: Cambridge University Press, 2000.

Ezell, Margaret. *The Patriarch's Wife: Literary Evidence and the History of the Family*. Chapel Hill: University of North Carolina Press, 1987.

Filmer, Robert. "Observations Concerning the Original of Government." In *Sir*

*Robert Filmer: Patriarcha and Other Writings,* edited by Johann P. Sommerville. Cambridge: Cambridge University Press, 1991.

———. *Sir Robert Filmer: Patriarcha and Other Writings.* Edited by Johann P. Sommerville. Cambridge: Cambridge University Press, 1991.

Fissell, Mary. "Gender and Generation: Representing Reproduction in Early Modern England." *Gender and History* 7. no. 3 (1995): 433–56.

———. "Hairy Women and Naked Truths: Gender and the Politics of Knowledge in *Aristotle's Masterpiece." William and Mary Quarterly,* 3rd ser., 60, no.1 (January 2003): 43–74.

———. "Making a Masterpiece: The *Aristotle* Texts in Medical Culture." In *Right Living: An Anglo-American Tradition of Self-Help Medicine and Hygiene,* edited by Charles E. Rosenberg. Baltimore: Johns Hopkins University Press, 2003.

———. "Readers, Texts, and Contexts: Vernacular Medical Works in Early Modern England." In *The Popularization of Medicine, 1650–1850,* edited by Roy Porter. London: Routledge, 1992.

———. *Vernacular Bodies: The Politics of Reproduction in Early Modern England.* Oxford: Oxford University Press, 2004.

Flanagan, Owen. *The Problem of the Soul: Two Visions of Mind and How to Reconcile Them.* New York: Basic Books, 2002.

———. *The Science of the Mind.* 2nd ed. Cambridge, Mass.: MIT Press, 1991.

Fleck, Ludwik. *Genesis and Development of a Scientific Fact.* Translated by Fred Bradley and Thaddeus J. Trenn. Chicago: University of Chicago Press, 1979.

———. "On the Crisis of 'Reality.'" In *Cognition and Fact: Materials on Ludwik Fleck,* edited by Robert S. Cohen and Thomas Schnelle. Dordrecht: D. Reidel, 1986.

Flemming, Rebecca. *Medicine and the Making of Roman Women: Gender, Nature, and Authority from Celsus to Galen.* Oxford: Oxford University Press, 2000.

Floyd-Wilson, Mary. *English Ethnicity and Race in Early Modern Drama.* Cambridge: Cambridge University Press, 2003.

Forrester, John. "The Marvellous Network and the History of Enquiry into its Function." *Journal of the History of Medicine and Allied Sciences* 57, no. 2 (2002): 198–217.

Fouke, Daniel C. "Mechanical and 'Organical' Models in Seventeenth-Century Explanations of Biological Reproduction." *Science in Context* 3, no. 2 (Autumn 1989): 366–81.

French, Roger. *Medicine before Science: The Rational and Learned Doctor from the Middle Ages to the Enlightenment.* Cambridge: Cambridge University Press, 2003.

Fuchs, Thomas. *The Mechanization of the Heart: Harvey and Descartes.* Translated by Marjorie Grene. Rochester: University of Rochester Press, 2001.

Furdell, Elizabeth. *Publishing and Medicine in Early Modern England.* Rochester: University of Rochester Press, 2002.

Galen. *On the Doctrines of Hippocrates and Plato.* Edited, translated, and with a commentary by Phillip De Lacy. 3 vols. Berlin: Akademie-Verlag, 1978–1984.

———. *On the Natural Faculties.* Edited and translated by Arthur John Brock. London: Hienemann, 1916.

———. *On the Usefulness of the Parts of the Body.* Translated by Margaret Tallmadge May. 2 vols. Ithaca: Cornell University Press, 1968.

———. *Opera Omnia*. Edited by Karl Gottlob Kühn and Friedrich Wilhelm Assmann. 22 vols. Leipzig: C. Cnobloch, 1821–1833.

———. *Selected Works*. Translated by P. N. Singer. Oxford: Oxford University Press, 1997.

García-Ballester, Luis. *Galen and Galenism: Theory and Medical Practice from Antiquity to the European Renaissance*. Burlington, VT: Ashgate, 2002.

———. "Soul and Body: Disease of the Soul and Disease of the Body in Galen's Medical Thought." In *Le opere psicologiche di Galeno*, edited by P. Manuli and M. Vegetti. Naples: Bibliopolis, 1988.

Gasking, Elizabeth. *Investigations into Generation, 1651–1828*. London: Hutchinson, 1967.

Geertz, Clifford. "From the Native's Point of View: On the Nature of Anthropological Understanding." In *Interpretive Social Science: a Reader*, edited by R. Rabinow and W. M. Sullivan. Berkeley: University of California Press, 1979.

Giffard, William. *Cases in Midwifery*. Edited by Edward Hody, MD. London: B. Motte and T. Wotton, 1734.

Gowing, Laura. *Common Bodies: Women, Touch, and Power in Seventeenth-Century England*. New Haven: Yale University Press, 2003.

Green, Monica. "'From Diseases of Women' to 'Secrets of Women': The Transformation of Gynecological Literature in the Later Middle Ages." *Journal of Medieval and Early Modern Studies* 30, no. 1 (2000): 5–39.

———. "Obstetrical and Gynaecological Texts in Middle English." *Studies in the Age of Chaucer* 14 (1992): 53–88.

Greenblatt, Stephen. *Renaissance Self-Fashioning: From More to Shakespeare*. Chicago: Chicago University Press, 1980.

Grosz, Elizabeth. *Volatile Bodies: Toward a Corporeal Feminism*. Bloomington, IN: Indiana University Press, 1994.

Grundy, Isobel. "Sarah Stone: Enlightenment Midwife." In *Medicine in the Enlightenment*, edited by Roy Porter. Amsterdam: Rodopi, 1995.

Guerrini, Anita. "The Burden of Procreation: Women and Preformation in the Works of George Garden and George Cheyne." In *Science and Medicine in the Scottish Enlightenment*, edited by Charles W. J. Withers and Paul Woods. East Linton: Tuckwell Press, 2002.

———. *Obesity and Depression in the Enlightenment: The Life and Times of George Cheyne*. Norman, OK: University of Oklahoma Press, 2000.

Guillemeau, Jacques. *Child-birth; or, The Happy Deliuerie of Women*. London: A. Hatfield, 1612.

Hankinson, R. James. "Actions and Passions: Affection, Emotion, and Moral Self-Management in Galen's Philosophical Psychology." In *Passions and Perceptions: Studies in Hellenistic Philosophy of Mind*, edited by Jacques Brunschwig and Martha C. Nussbaum. Cambridge: Cambridge University Press, 1993.

———. "Galen's Anatomy of the Soul." *Phronesis* 26, no. 2 (1991): 197–233.

Haraway, Donna J. *Simians, Cyborgs, and Women: the Reinvention of Nature*. New York: Routledge, 1991.

Harvey, Elizabeth. "Sensational Bodies, Consenting Organs: Helkiah Crooke's Incorporation of Spenser." *Spenser Studies: A Renaissance Poetry Annual* 18 (2003): 295–314.

Harvey, William. *The Anatomical Exercises of Dr. William Harvey, De Motu Cordis* 1628: *De Circulatione Sanguinis* 1649: *The First English Text of* 1653. Edited by Geoffrey Keynes. London: Nonesuch, 1928.

———. *Anatomical Exercises on the Generation of Animals.* In *The Works of William Harvey*, translated by Robert Willis. 145–589. London: Sydenham Society, 1847.

———. *Anatomical Exercitations, Concerning the Generation of Living Creatures.* London: James Young, 1653.

Hayles, N. Katherine. *How We Became Posthuman: Virtual Bodies in Cybernetics, Literature, and Informatics.* Chicago: University of Chicago Press, 1999.

Henderson, Andrea. "Doll-Machines and Butcher-Shop Meat: Models of Childbirth in the Early Stages of Industrial Capitalism." *Genders* 12 (Winter, 1991): 100–19.

Highmore, Nathaniel. *The History of Generation.* London: John Martin, 1651.

Hill, Christopher. "William Harvey and the Idea of Monarchy." In *The Intellectual Revolution of the Seventeenth Century*, edited by Charles Webster. London: Routledge, 1974.

Hillman, David, and Carla Mazzio, eds. *The Body in Parts: Fantasies of Corporeality in Early Modern Europe.* New York: Routledge, 1997.

Hobbes, Thomas. *Leviathan.* Edited by C. B. Macpherson. Harmondsworth, Middlesex: Penguin Books, 1968.

———. *Man and Citizen.* Edited by Bernard Gert. Gloucester, Mass.: Peter Smith, 1978.

Horowitz, Maryanne Cline. "The 'Science' of Embryology before the Discovery of the Ovum." In *Connecting Spheres: Women in the Western World, 1500–Present*, edited by Marilyn Boxer and Jean Quataert. New York: Oxford University Press, 1987.

Houtzager, H. L. "Hendrik van Deventer." In *European Journal of Obstetrics, Gynaecology and Reproductive Biology* 21 (1986): 263–70.

Huet, Marie-Hélène. *Monstrous Imagination.* Cambridge, Mass.: Harvard University Press, 1993.

Hughes, Ann. "Gender and Politics in Leveller Literature." In *Political Culture and Cultural Politics in Early Modern England*, edited by Susan Amussen and Mark Kishlansky. Manchester: Manchester University Press, 1995.

Jacquart, Danielle, and Claude Thomasset. *Sexuality and Medicine in the Middle Ages.* Cambridge: Polity Press, 1988.

Johnston, John. "A Future for Autonomous Agents: Machinic *Merkwelten* and Artificial Evolution." *Configurations* 10, no. 3 (2002): 473–517.

Jonas, Richard, trans. *The Byrth of Mankynde, newly translated out of Laten into Englysshe.* London: Thomas Raynalde, 1540.

Jordanova, Ludmilla. "Gender, Generation, and Science: William Hunter's Obstetrical Atlas." In *William Hunter and the Eighteenth-Century Medical World*, edited by W. F. Bynum and Roy Porter. Cambridge: Cambridge University Press, 1985.

Jorden, Edward. *A Briefe Discourse of a Disease Called the Suffocation of the Womb.* London: John Windet, 1603.

Keller, Eve. "Mrs. Jane Sharp: Midwifery and the Critique of Medical Knowledge in Seventeenth-Century England." *Women's Writing* 2, no. 2 (1995): 101–11.

Keller, Evelyn Fox. "Baconian Science: A Hermaphroditic Birth." *Philosophical Forum* 11 (1980): 299–308.

Keynes, Geoffrey. *The Life of William Harvey*. Oxford: Clarendon Press, 1966.

King, Helen. "'As if None Understood the Art that Cannot Understand Greek': The Education of Midwives in Seventeenth-Century England." In *The History of Medical Education in Britain*, edited by Vivian Nutton and Roy Porter. Amsterdam: Rodopi, 1995.

———. "Green Sickness: Hippocrates, Galen, and the Origins of the 'Disease of Virgins.'" *International Journal of the Classical Tradition* 2 (1996): 372–87.

———. "Once upon a Text: the Hippocratic Origins of Hysteria." In *Hysteria Beyond Freud*, edited by Sander L. Gilman, Helen King, Roy Porter, G. S. Rousseau, and Elaine Showalter. Berkeley: University of California Press, 1993.

———. "The Power of Paternity: The Father of Medicine Meets the Prince of Physicians." In *Reinventing Hippocrates*, edited by David Cantor. Burlington, VT: Ashgate, 2002.

Kirkpatrick, Robin. *The European Renaissance, 1400–1600*. London: Longman, 2002.

Kuhn, Thomas. *The Structure of Scientific Revolutions*. Chicago: Chicago University Press, 1962.

Kuriyama, Shigehisa. *The Expressiveness of the Body and the Divergence of Greek and Chinese Medicine*. New York: Zone Books, 1999.

Laqueur, Thomas. *Making Sex: Body and Gender from the Greeks to Freud*. Cambridge, Mass.: Harvard University Press, 1990.

Latour, Bruno. *We Have Never Been Modern*. Translated by Catherine Porter. Cambridge: Harvard University Press, 1993.

———. "Why Has Critique Run out of Steam? From Matters of Fact to Matters of Concern." *Critical Inquiry* 30, no. 2 (Winter, 2004): 225–48.

MacDonald, Michael. *Witchcraft and Hysteria in Elizabethan London: Edward Jorden and the Mary Glover Case*. London: Tavistock/Routledge, 1991.

MacLean, Ian. *The Renaissance Notion of Woman: a Study in the Fortunes of Scholasticism and Medical Science in European Intellectual Life*. Cambridge: Cambridge University Press, 1980.

MacPherson, C. B. *The Political Theory of Possessive Individualism: Hobbes to Locke*. Oxford: Clarendon Press, 1962.

Maddison, Frederick Romeril, Margaret Pelling, and Charles Webster, eds. *Essays on the Life and Work of Thomas Linacre, c. 1460–1524*. Oxford: Clarendon Press, 1977.

Martenson, Robert. "The Transformation of Eve: Women's Bodies, Medicine, and Culture in Early Modern England." In *Sexual Knowledge, Sexual Science: The History of Attitudes to Sexuality*, edited by Roy Porter and Mikulas Teich. Cambridge: Cambridge University Press, 1997.

Martin, John Jeffries. *Myths of Renaissance Individualism*. New York: Palgrave Macmillan, 2004.

Matson, Wallace I. "Why Isn't the Mind-Body Problem Ancient?" In *Mind, Matter, and Method: Essays in Philosophy and Science in Honor of Herbert Feigl*, edited by Paul Feyerabend and Grover Maxwell. Minneapolis: University of Minnesota Press, 1966.

Maubray, John. *The Female Physician*. London: James Holland, 1724.

Maus, Katherine. *Inwardness and Theater in the English Renaissance*. Chicago: University of Chicago Press, 1995.

Maxwell, John. *Sacro-Santa Regnum Majestas; or, The Sacred and Royall Prerogative of Christian Kings*. Oxford: Henry Hall, 1644.

McLaren, Angus. *Reproductive Rituals: the Perception of Fertility in England from the Sixteenth to the Nineteenth Century*. London: Methuen, 1984.

Mears, Martha. *The Pupil of Nature*. London: L. Lichfield, 1797.

Meyer, A. W. *An Analysis of the "De generatione" of William Harvey*. Stanford: Stanford University Press, 1936.

Milton, John. *Paradise Lost*, in *John Milton: Complete Poems and Major Prose*, edited by Merritt Y. Hughes. New York: Odyssey Press, 1957.

Mitchell, William. *Me ++: The Cyborg Self and the Networked City*. Cambridge, Mass.: MIT Press, 2003.

Moravec, Hans P. *Mind Children: The Future of Robot and Human Intelligence*. Cambridge, Mass.: Harvard University Press, 1988.

———. *Robot: Mere Machine to Transcendent Mind*. New York: Oxford University Press, 1999.

Müller-Sievers, Helmut. *Self-Generation: Biology, Philosophy, and Literature around 1800*. Stanford: Stanford University Press, 1997.

Nagel, Thomas. "What Is It Like to Be a Bat?" In *Mortal Questions*. Cambridge: Cambridge University Press, 1979.

Nagy, Doreen G. *Popular Medicine in Seventeenth-Century England*. Bowling Green, OH: Bowling Green State University Popular Press, 1988.

Needham, Joseph. *A History of Embryology*. 1957. Reprint, New York: Arno Press, 1975.

Newman, Karen. *Fetal Positions: Individualism, Science, Visuality*. Stanford: Stanford University Press, 1996.

Nicolson, Malcolm. "The Art of Diagnosis: Medicine and the Five Senses." In *Companion Encyclopedia of the History of Medicine*, edited by W. F. Bynum and Roy Porter. 2:801–25. London: Routledge, 1993.

Nihell, Elizabeth. *A Treatise on the Art of Midwifery*. London: A. Morely, 1760.

Nutton, Vivan, ed. *Galen: Problems and Prospects*. London: Wellcome Institute for the History of Medicine, 1981.

———. "Hippocrates in the Renaissance." In *Die Hippokratischen Epidemien: Theorie—Praxis—Tradition: Verhandlungen des Ve Colloque International Hippocratique, Sudhoffs Archiv Beiheft* 27 (1989): 420–39.

———. *John Caius and the Manuscripts of Galen*. Cambridge: Cambridge Philological Society, 1987.

———. "The Seeds of Disease: An Explanation of Contagion and Infection from the Greeks to the Renaissance." *Medical History* 27 (1983): 1–34.

———, ed. *The Unknown Galen*. Bulletin of the Institute of Classical Studies 77. London: Institute of Classical Studies, School of Advanced Studies, University of London, 2002.

Nyquist, Mary. "The Genesis of Gendered Subjectivity in the Divorce Tracts and in *Paradise Lost*." In *Re-Membering Milton: Essays on the Texts and Traditions*, edited by Mary Nyquist and Margaret Furgeson. New York: Methuen, 1987.

O'Malley, Charles David. *English Medical Humanists, Thomas Linacre and John*

*Caius*. Lawrence; University of Kansas Press, 1965.

———. "Helkiah Crooke, M.D., P.R.C.P., 1576–1648." *Bulletin of the History of Medicine* 42, no. 1 (1968): 1–18.

Oppenheimer, Jane. *Essays in the History of Embryology and Biology*. Cambridge, Mass.: MIT Press, 1967.

Pagel, Walter. *William Harvey's Biological Ideas: Selected Aspects and Historical Background*. New York: Hafner, 1967.

———. *New Light on William Harvey*. Basel: Karger, 1978.

Park, Katherine, and Robert Nye. "Destiny is Anatomy." *The New Republic* 18 February, 1991, 53–57.

Parker, Patricia. "Rude Mechanicals." In *Subject and Object in Renaissance Culture*, edited by Margreta de Grazia, Maureen Quilligan, and Peter Stallybrass. Cambridge: Cambridge University Press, 1996.

Paster, Gail Kern. *The Body Embarrassed: Drama and the Disciplines of Shame in Early Modern England*. Ithaca: Cornell University Press, 1993.

———. *Humoring the Body: Emotions and the Shakespearean Stage*. Chicago: University of Chicago Press, 2004.

———, Katherine Rowe, and Mary Floyd-Wilson, eds. *Reading the Early Modern Passions: Essays in the Cultural History of Emotion*. Philadelphia: University of Pennsylvania Press, 2004.

Pateman, Carole. *The Disorder of Women: Democracy, Feminism, and Political Theory*. Stanford: Stanford University Press, 1989.

———. "'God Hath Ordained to Man a Helper': Hobbes, Patriarchy, and Conjugal Right." In *Feminist Interpretations and Political Theory*, edited by Mary Lyndon Shanley and Carole Pateman. Cambridge: Polity Press, 1990.

———. *The Sexual Contract*. Stanford: Stanford University Press, 1988.

Pelling, Margaret. *The Common Lot: Sickness, Medical Occupations and the Urban Poor in Early Modern England*. London: Longman, 1988.

———. "Contagion/Germ Theory/Specificity." In *Companion Encyclopedia of the History of Medicine*, edited by W. F. Bynum and Roy Porter. 1:309–34. London: Routledge, 1993.

———. *Medical Conflicts in Early Modern London: Patronage, Physicians, and Irregular Practitioners 1550–1640*. Oxford: Oxford University Press, 2003.

*Philosophical Transactions of the Royal Society*. London: C. Davis, Printer to the Royal Society of London, 1665–1775.

Pinto-Carreia, Clara. *The Ovary of Eve: Egg and Sperm and Preformation*. Chicago: University of Chicago Press, 1997.

Pollack, Linda. "Embarking on a Rough Passage: The Experience of Pregnancy in Early-Modern Society." In *Women as Mothers in Pre-Industrial England: Essays in Memory of Dorothy McLaren*, edited by Valerie Fildes. London: Routledge, 1990.

———. "Childbearing and Female Bonding in Early Modern England." *Social History* 22, no. 3 (1997): 286–306.

Porter, Dorothy, and Roy Porter. *Patient's Progress: Doctors and Doctoring in 18th-Century England*. Stanford: Stanford University Press, 1989.

Porter, Roy, ed. *Medicine and the Enlightenment*. Amsterdam: Rodopi, 1995.

———. *Patients and Practitioners: Lay Perceptions of Medicine in Pre-Industrial Society*. Cambridge: Cambridge University Press, 1985.

———. "The Patient's View: Doing Medical History from Below." *Theory and Society* 14 (1985): 175–98.

———, ed. *The Popularization of Medicine, 1650–1750.* London: Routledge, 1992.

———, ed. *Rewriting the Self: Histories from the Renaissance to the Present.* London: Routledge, 1997.

———. "The Rise of Physical Examination." In *Medicine and the Five Senses*, edited by W. F. Bynum and Roy Porter. Cambridge: Cambridge University Press, 1993.

———. "A Touch of Danger: The Man-Midwife as Sexual Predator." In *Sexual Underworlds of the Enlightenment*, edited by G. S. Rousseau and Roy Porter. 206–32. Manchester: Manchester University Press, 1987.

———, and Dorothy Porter, eds. *In Sickness and in Health: The British Experience 1650–1850.* London: Fourth Estate, 1988.

———, and Dorothy Porter, eds. *Patient's Progress: Sickness, Health and Medical Care in England, 1650–1850.* London: Polity Press, 1989.

———, and Lesley Hall. *The Facts of Life: The Creation of Sexual Knowledge in Britain, 1650–1950.* New Haven: Yale University Press, 1995.

Poynter, F. N. L. "Nicholas Culpeper and his Books." *Journal of the History of Medicine* 17 (1962): 152–67.

———. "Nicholas Culpeper and the Paracelsians." In *Science, Medicine, and Society in the Renaissance: Essays to Honor Walter Pagel*, edited by Allen G. Debus.1: 201–20. New York: American Elsevier Press, 1972.

Pyle, A. J. "Animal Generation and the Mechanical Philosophy: Some Light on the Role of Biology in the Scientific Revolution." *History and Philosophy of the Life Sciences* 9 (1987): 225–54.

Ramachandran, V. S., and Sandra Blakeslee. *Phantoms in the Brain: Probing the Mysteries of the Human Mind.* New York: William Morrow, 1998.

Rawcliffe, Carole. *Medicine and Society in Later Medieval England.* Phoenix Mill: Sutton Publishing, 1997.

Raynalde, Thomas, trans. *The Byrth of Mankynde*, by Eucharius Rösslin. London: Thomas Raynalde, 1545.

Reiser, S. J. *Medicine and the Reign of Technology.* Cambridge: Cambridge University Press, 1978.

Reiss, Timothy J. *Mirages of the Selfe: Patterns of Personhood in Ancient and Early Modern Europe.* Stanford: Stanford University Press, 2003.

Riddle, John M. *Contraception and Abortion from the Ancient World to the Renaissance.* Cambridge, Mass.: Harvard University Press, 1992.

Riverius, Lazarus. *The Practice of Physicke.* Translated by Nicholas Culpeper, Abdiah Cole, and William Rowland. London: George Sawbridge, 1678.

Rocca, Julius. *Galen on the Brain: Anatomical Knowledge and Physiological Speculation in the Second Century.* Leiden, Boston: Brill, 2003.

Roe, Shirley. *Matter, Life, and Generation: Eighteenth-Century Embryology and the Haller-Wolff Debate.* Cambridge: Cambridge University Press, 1981.

Roger, Jacques. *Les sciences de la vie dans la pensée française du XVIIIc siècle: la génération des animaux de Descartes à l'encyclopédie.* Paris: Armand Collin, 1963.

Rogers, John. *The Matter of Revolution:*

*Science, Poetry, and Politics in the Age of Milton.* Ithaca: Cornell University Press, 1996.

Rösslin, Eucharius. *The Byrth of Mankynde,* Translated by Richard Jonas. London: Thomas Raynalde, 1540.

———. *The Byrth of Mankynde,* Translated by Thomas Raynalde. London: Thomas Raynalde, 1545.

Rousseau, G. S. "'A Strange Pathology': Hysteria in the Early Modern World, 1500–1800." In *Hysteria Beyond Freud,* edited by Sander Gilman, Helen King, Roy Porter, G. S. Rousseau, and Elaine Showalter. Berkeley: University of California Press, 1993.

Rousseau, G. S., and Roy Porter. "Introduction: Toward a Natural History of Mind and Body." In *The Languages of Psyche: Mind and Body in Enlightenment Thought: Clark Library Lectures, 1985–1986,* edited by G. S. Rousseau. Berkeley: University of California Press, 1990.

Rueff, Jacob. *De Conceptu et Generatione Homins.* London: E. Griffin. 1637 [1554].

Ruestow, Edward. "Leeuwenhoek's Perception of the Spermatozoa." *Journal of the History of Biology* 6, no. 2 (1983): 185–224.

Russell, K. F. "A Checklist of Medical Books Published in English before 1600." *Bulletin of the History of Medicine* 21 (1947): 922–58.

Sadler, John. *The Sicke Womans Private Looking-Glasse.* London: Anne Griffin, 1636.

Sawday, Jonathan. *The Body Emblazoned: Dissection and the Human Body in Renaissance Culture.* London, New York: Routledge, 1995.

———. "The Fate of Marsyas: Dissecting the Renaissance Body." In *Renaissance Bodies: The Human Figure in English Culture c. 1540–1660,* edited by Lucy Gent and Nigel Llewellyn. London: Reaktion, 1990.

———. "Self and Selfhood in the Seventeenth Century." In *Rewriting the Self: Histories from the Renaissance to the Present,* edited by Roy Porter. London: Routledge, 1997.

Schiebinger, Londa. *The Mind Has No Sex?: Women in the Origins of Modern Science.* Cambridge, Mass.: Harvard University Press, 1989.

Schierbeck, A. *Jan Swammerdam. 12 February 1637–17 February 1680. His Life and Works.* Amsterdam: Swets Zeitlinger, 1967.

Schleiner, Winfried. "Early Modern Controversies about the One-Sex Model." *Renaissance Quarterly* 53, no.1 (2000): 180–91.

Schochet, Gordon J. *Patriarchalism in Political Thought: The Authoritarian Family and Political Speculation and Attitudes, Especially in Seventeenth-Century England.* New York: Basic Books, 1975.

———. "The Significant Sounds of Silence: the Absence of Women from the Political Thought of Sir Robert Filmer and John Locke (or, 'Why Can't a Woman be More Like a Man?')." In *Women Writers and the Early Modern British Political Tradition,* edited by Hilda Smith. Cambridge: Cambridge University Press, 1998.

Schoenfeldt, Michael C. *Bodies and Selves in Early Modern England: Physiology and Inwardness in Spenser, Shakespeare, Herbert, and Milton.* Cambridge: Cambridge University Press, 1999.

Securis, John. *A Detection and Querimonie of*

the Daily Enormities and Abuses Comitted in Physick. London: T. Marsh, 1566.

Sermon, William. The Ladies Companion, or, The English Midwife. London: E. Thomas, 1671.

Shanley, Mary. "Marriage Contract and Social Contract in Seventeenth-Century Political Thought." Western Political Quarterly 32 (1979): 79–91.

Sharp, Jane. The Midwives Book, or, the Whole Art of Midwifry Discovered. 1671. Edited by Elaine Hobby. New York: Oxford University Press, 1999.

Shoemaker, Robert Brink. Gender in English Society, 1650–1850: The Emergence of Separate Spheres? London: Longman, 1998.

Shorter, Edward. Women's Bodies: A Social History of Women's Encounter with Health, Ill-Health and Medicine. New Brunswick, NJ: Transaction Publications, 1991.

Siraisi, Nancy G. Medieval and Early Renaissance Medicine: An Introduction to Knowledge and Practice. Chicago: University of Chicago Press, 1990.

Slack, Paul. "Mirrors of Health and Treasures of Poor Men: the Uses of Vernacular Medical Literature of Tudor England." In Health, Medicine, and Mortality in the Sixteenth Century, edited by C. Webster. Cambridge: Cambridge University Press, 1979.

Smith, Roger. "Self-Reflection and the Self." In Rewriting the Self: Histories from the Renaissance to the Present, edited by Roy Porter. London: Routledge, 1997.

Speert, Harold. Iconographia Gyniatrica: A Pictorial History of Gynecology and Obstetrics. Philadelphia: F. A. Davis, 1973.

Stine, Jennifer. "Opening Closets: The Discovery of Household Medicine in Early Modern England." PhD diss., Stanford, 1996.

Stolberg, Michael. "A Woman Down to Her Bones: The Anatomy of Sexual Difference in the Sixteenth and Early Seventeenth Centuries." Isis 94, no. 2 (2003): 274–99.

Stone, Sarah. A Complete Practice of Midwifery. London: T. Cooper, 1737.

Sudell, Nicholas. Mulierum Amicus; or, the Woman's Friend. London: J. Hancock, 1666.

Sutton, John. Philosophy and Memory Traces: Descartes to Connectionism. Cambridge: Cambridge University Press, 1998.

Symcotts, John. A Seventeenth-Century Doctor and His Patients: John Symcotts, 1592?–1662. Edited by F. N. L Poynter and W. J. Bishop. Publications of the Bedfordshire Historical Record Society 31. Streatley: Bedfordshire Publication Society, 1951.

Taylor, Charles. Sources of the Self: The Making of Modern Identity. Cambridge, Mass.: Harvard University Press, 1989.

Temkin, Owsei. Galenism: Rise and Decline of a Medical Philosophy. Ithaca: Cornell University Press, 1973.

Thacker, Eugene. "Data Made Flesh: Biotechnology and the Discourse of the Posthuman." Cultural Critique 53 (2003): 72–97.

Thulesius, Olav. Nicholas Culpeper, English Physician and Astrologer. New York: St. Martin's Press, 1992.

Toulmin, Estephen. "Ludwik Fleck and the Historical Interpretation of Science." In Cognition and Fact: Materials on Ludwik Fleck, edited by R. S. Cohen and T. Schnelle. Dordrecht: D. Reidel, 1986.

Traub, Valerie. "Gendering Mortality in Early Modern Anatomies." In Feminist Readings of Early Modern Culture: Emerging Subjects, edited by Valerie Traub,

M. Lindsay Kaplan, and Dympna Callaghan. Cambridge: Cambridge University Press, 1996.

———. *The Renaissance of Lesbianism in Early Modern England*. Cambridge: Cambridge University Press, 2002.

Tuana, Nancy. *The Less Noble Sex: Scientific, Religious, and Philosophical Conceptions of Woman's Nature*. Bloomington, IN: Indiana University Press, 1993.

van Deventer, Henry. *The Art of Midwifery Improv'd*. Translated by Robert Samber. London: E. Curll, J. Pemberton, and W. Taylor, 1716.

Varela, Francisco J., Evan Thompson, and Eleanor Rosch. *The Embodied Mind: Cognitive Science and Human Experience*. Cambridge, Mass.: MIT Press, 1991.

Vicary, Thomas. *Anatomie of the Bodie of Man*. 1548. Edited by Frederick James Furnivall and Percy Furnivall. EETS ES 53. London: Oxford University Press, 1930.

Voss, Stephen. "Descartes: Heart and Soul." In *Pysche and Soma: Physicians and metaphysicians on the mind-body problem from Antiquity to Enlightenment*, edited by John P. Wright and Paul Potter. Oxford: Clarendon Press, 2000.

Warhaft, Sidney, ed. *Francis Bacon: A Selection of his Works*. Indianapolis: Bobbs-Merrill Educational Publishing, 1965.

Wear, Andrew. "Galen in the Renaissance." In *Galen: Problems and Prospects*, edited by Vivian Nutton. 229-63. London: Wellcome Institute for the History of Medicine, 1981.

———. *Knowledge and Practice in Early Modern English Medicine, 1550–1680*. Cambridge: Cambridge University Press, 2000.

———. "Popularization of Medicine in Early Modern England." In *The Popularization of Medicine 1650–1750*, edited by Roy Porter. London: Routledge, 1992.

Webster, Charles. *The Great Instauration: Science, Medicine, and Reform, 1626–1660*. London: Duckworth, 1975.

Weil, Rachel J. *Political Passions: Gender, the Family, and Political Argument in England, 1680–1714*. Manchester: Manchester University Press, 1999.

Whately, William. *A Bride-Bush or a Vvedding Sermon*. London: William Iaggard, 1617.

Whitteridge, Gweneth. "William Harvey: A Royalist and No Parliamentarian." In *The Intellectual Revolution of the Seventeenth Century*, edited by Charles Webster. London: Routledge, 1974.

Willughby, Percival. *Observations in Midwifery*. 1863. Facsimile reprint with an introduction by John L. Thornton. Wakefield: S. R. Publishers, 1972.

Wilson, Adrian. "The Ceremony of Childbirth and its Interpretation." In *Women as Mothers in Pre-Industrial England: Essays in Memory of Dorothy McLaren*, edited by Valerie Fildes. London: Routledge, 1990.

———. *The Making of Man-Midwifery: Childbirth in England, 1660–1770*. Cambridge, Mass.: Harvard University Press, 1995.

———. "A Memorial of Eleanor Willughby, a Seventeenth-Century Midwife." In *Women, Science and Medicine 1500–1700: Mothers and Sisters of the Royal Society*, edited by Lynette Hunter and Sarah Hutton. Phoenix Mill: Sutton Publishing, 1997.

———. "Participant versus Patient: Seventeenth-Century Childbirth from the Mother's Point of View." In *Patients and Practitioners: Lay Perceptions of Medicine in Pre-Industrial Society*, edited by Roy Porter. Cambridge: Cambridge University Press, 1986.

Wilson, Elizabeth. *Neural Geographies: Feminism and the Microstructure of Cognition*. London: Routledge, 1998.

———. *Psychosomatic: Feminism and the Neurological Body*. Durham, NC: Duke University Press, 2004.

Wiseman, Susan. "'Adam, the Father of All Flesh': Porno-Political Rhetoric and Political Theory in and After the English Civil War." In *Pamphlet Wars: Prose in the English Revolution*, edited by James Holstun. London: Frank Cass, 1992.

Wolfe, Cary. *Animal Rites: American Culture, the Discourse of Species, and Posthumanist Theory*. Chicago: University of Chicago Press, 2003.

Wolveridge, James. *Speculum matricis hybernicum; or, the Irish Midwives Handmaid*. London: E. Okes, 1670.

Wright, John P. "Hysteria and Mechanical Man." *Journal of the History of Ideas* 41, no. 2 (1980): 233–47.

———, and Paul Potter, eds. *Psyche and Soma: Physicians and Metaphysicians on the Mind-Body Problem from Antiquity to Enlightenment*. Oxford: Clarendon Press, 2000.

Yolton, John W. *Thinking Matter: Materialism in Eighteenth-Century Britain*. Minneapolis: University of Minnesota Press, 1983.

# INDEX

*Page numbers in italics refer to illustrations*